RIDING AND ROADCRAFT

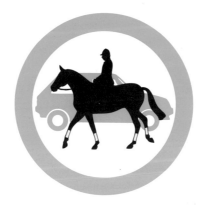

Riding and Road Safety Manual

9TH EDITION

THE BRITISH HORSE SOCIETY

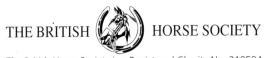

THE BRITISH HORSE SOCIETY

The British Horse Society is a Registered Charity No. 210504

ACKNOWLEDGEMENTS

The Policy Committee wishes to thank: Mr B.A.C. Hughes and VAG (UK) Ltd for their illustrations; for illustrations in the Falls and Injuries section – full information appears in the First Aid Manual from which information is reproduced by kind permission of St John Ambulance, St Andrew's Ambulance Association and British Red Cross, published by Dorling Kindersley price £8.99, and The Pony Club; Dr J.M.H. Lloyd-Parry MA, MB, BChir., Honorary Medical Adviser to the Horse Trials Group and Vice-chairman of the Safety Policy Committee, for the section on Falls and Injuries; Mrs S. Walrond and Lt Col. D.S. Barker Simson, former Chairman of the Safety Policy Committee, for their work on the driving section, reproduced in this from the previous edition; Miss Ann C. Norris, originator of Driving logo illustration; the Side-Saddle Association for their advice on the side-saddle section; Police Constable D. Moss-Norbury of Thames Valley Police; Crown copyright is reproduced with the permission of the Controller of HMSO; the Chairman of the Safety Policy Committee, Mrs Sheila Berry and the National Safety Officer, Mrs Lesley Billingham for their editorial directions; Miss A.L. Smith, Mrs J. Mann and Mrs J. Hughes – Manual Working Party for the 8th Edition on which the 9th Edition is based together with original notes for previous editions made by Denis Colton, former Chief Inspector, Metropolitan Mounted Branch.

Published by The British Horse Society for the Safety Policy Committee (Road Safety Division), British Equestrian Centre, Stoneleigh Park, Kenilworth, Warwickshire, CV8 2LR.

© British Horse Society, 1995.

First published in 1976 as *Ride Safely*.

Revised in 1984 as *Ride and Drive Safely*.

Revised in 1986 as *Riding and Roadcraft*, except 7th edition published 1989 and revised 1990.

Eighth edition, 1993.

Ninth edition, 1995, reprinted 1997.

British Library Cataloguing in Publication Data
A catalogue record for this book is available from the British Library.

ISBN 1-872082-78-5

A contribution from sales of this publication is made to the British Horse Society's Road Safety Campaign Fund.

Cover design: Paul Saunders.
Text design: Phil Kay.

Produced by The Kenilworth Press Ltd, Addington, Buckingham, MK18 2JR
Printed by Westway Offset Ltd, Wembley.

CONTENTS

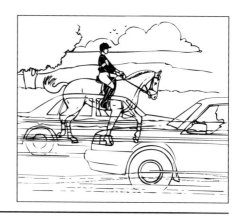
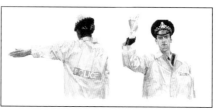
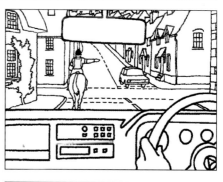
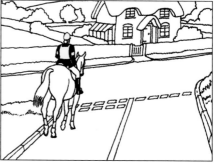

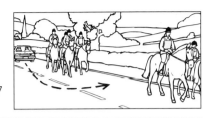

4. SIDE-SADDLE HORSE AND RIDER

5. FALLS AND INJURIES

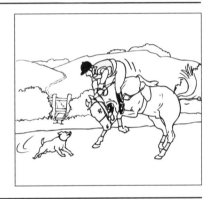

6. DRIVING HORSE-DRAWN VEHICLES

7. BHS RIDING AND ROAD SAFETY TEST

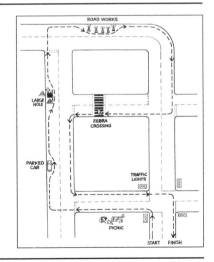

FOREWORD

I am delighted to welcome the ninth edition of this important manual from the British Horse Society. Horses are precious animals. Nobody wants to see them, or their riders, involved in road accidents. This manual will provide riders, whether novice or experienced, with invaluable information to help keep the roads safer for themselves, their horses, and other road users.

To avoid accidents to yourself or your horse I strongly recommend you to follow the Manual's excellent advice – not least that you should take the Riding and Road Safety Test.

Dr Brian Mawhinney
Secretary of State for Transport

INTRODUCTION

With the weight of today's traffic, everyone who uses any road is at risk. This is especially true when leading, riding or even driving a horse. The British Horse Society is involved in many spheres, but the safety of the horse and its rider or driver is paramount. This Manual is intended to help anyone who has to take a horse on the road. Experienced or otherwise, we can learn from the wise instruction found within these pages.

I implore you therefore, to read, mark, learn and inwardly digest this advice and to put it into practice whenever you are on the road with your horse. Don't forget: he is precious and so are you. Take care.

Edward Bonnor-Maurice
Chairman

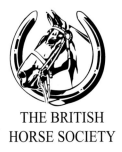

THE BRITISH
HORSE SOCIETY

AIM

The aim of this Manual is, in conjunction with the Highway Code, to promote responsible, considerate and courteous riding on the public highway by all riders, and through correct training to promote testing for the Society's Riding and Road Safety Test.

1. ARE YOU READY FOR THE ROAD?

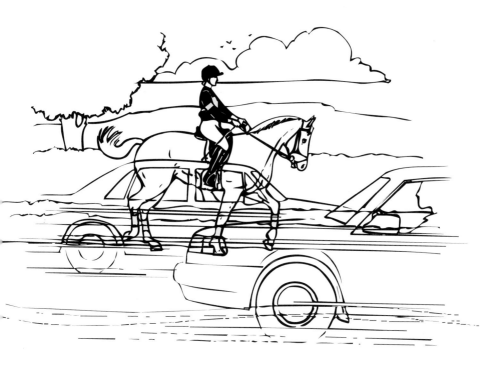

Highway Code: Rule 3 – Wear or carry something that will help you to be seen. Light-coloured, bright or fluorescent items will help in poor visibility. At night use reflective materials (e.g. reflective armbands and sashes) which can be seen in headlights up to three times as far away as non-reflective materials.

(See also Rules 219 and 224.)

BE SEEN TO BE SAFE

ALWAYS USE FLUORESCENT/REFLECTIVE LEG-BANDS, TABARDS AND HAT COVERS

How to prepare

(See Highway Code: Rules 216–224)

Highway Code: Rule 216 – Before you take a horse on to a road, make sure you can control it…

Before riding on the public highway, you should be a competent rider. Special training in the skills of roadcraft and a thorough understanding of the current edition of the Highway Code and its advice to all road users are necessary. The Highway Code is available at most bookshops. This Manual should be read in conjunction with the Highway Code.

To keep horses' hooves and shoes in good condition they should be regularly attended by the farrier. It is advisable to carry a folding hoof-pick, money for the telephone, string.

Consideration and courtesy

Good manners play an important part in roadcraft. Consideration and courtesy shown by horse riders to other road users helps foster good relations between them.

Always acknowledge acts of courtesy shown by other road users.

Insurance

Under certain circumstances a rider is likely to be considered liable if his horse/pony causes any harm to other people or to their property, and may be required to pay considerable damages. Riders and horse owners are therefore strongly advised to hold personal liability insurance. **This insurance cover is automatically extended to full members of the British Horse Society and members of the Pony Club.**

Novice or nervous horses

Highway Code: Rule 216 – If you think that your horse will be nervous of traffic, always ride with other, less-nervous horses.

A nervous or traffic-shy horse should go out on the road only in the company of a steady horse. Avoid main roads. Avoid peak traffic times.

Novice riders

Inexperienced riders should ride on the public highway in the company of an experienced rider. Avoid peak traffic times.

Young riders

Highway Code: Rule 7 – Most children under ten cannot judge how fast vehicles are going or how far away they are.

Parents and/or guardians are responsible for deciding at what age their children may ride on the road on their own.

All riders should leave details of their intended route and estimated time of return with a responsible person in the yard or at home.

By law children under the age of fourteen **MUST** wear an approved safety helmet.

Tack and equipment

Highway Code: Rule 217 – Make sure all tack fits well and is in good condition. Never ride a horse without a saddle or bridle.

When riding on the public highway, a saddle and bridle must always be used. When leading a horse, either mounted or dismounted, the led horse must always wear a bridle.

Ensure all tack is in good repair and that it fits correctly. Stitching and leather should be inspected regularly to ensure it is sound. Pliant tack adds to the comfort of the horse.

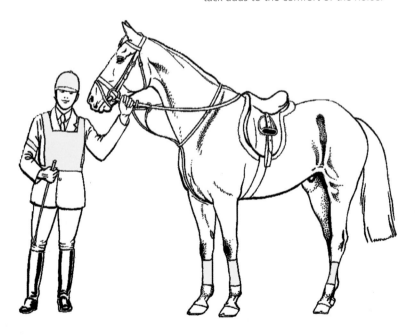

Ready for the road.

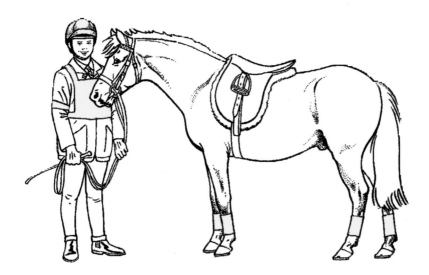

Be seen to be safe.

Great care should be taken to ensure that synthetic and adjustable saddles are correctly adjusted for comfort and fit.

> Highway Code: Rule 224 – Keep both feet in the stirrups…

Stirrup irons should be the correct size for the rider's foot, as a guide a minimum of 6mm (¼ inch) clearance on either side at the ball of the foot when in the stirrup.

It is inadvisable to use nickel stirrup irons or bits.

Stirrup leathers must easily release from stirrup bars. Never ride with stirrup bars up.

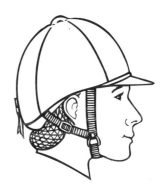

BS EN 1384 (97) and PAS 015 (94)

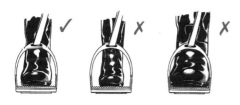

Hats

> Highway Code: Rule 218 – Wear an approved safety helmet and fasten it securely – children under the age of fourteen **MUST** do this.

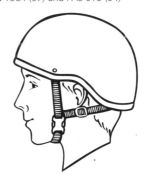

The BS EN 1384 (97) and the PAS 015 (94) (Product Approval Specification) are Kitemarked and recommended by the British Horse Society.

For maximum protection, headgear should conform to BS EN 1384 (97) or PAS 015 (94), with shock absorption to the bottom edge. These standards are acceptable for the BHS Riding and Road Safety Test.

The hat worn by the rider should be the rider's own hat and fit correctly. The hat should be secured with a minimum three-point harness. For *maximum* protection, the headgear should be Kitemarked and conform to PAS 015 (94) or BS EN 1384 (97) (the British version of the European standard) or to an at least equal standard.

Current recommendations of the British Horse Society are that hats to the standards PAS 015 (94) and BS EN 1384 (97) are worn, but equivalent standards such as ASTM (SEI) F1163 are considered acceptable – although it remains a matter of concern that the ventilation slashes allow the remote possibility of a penetration injury.

The hat must fit and be properly secured. It must be in good condition.
ALWAYS WEAR IT

From 30th June 1992, children under the age of fourteen years, must by law wear protective headgear whenever riding a horse on the road. Failure to do so may result in prosecution of the parent, employers or any other person supervising, or otherwise connected with, the minor.

The Horses (Protective Headgear for Young Riders) Regulations 1992.

Footwear

▌ Highway Code: Rule 218 – wear boots or shoes with hard soles and heels.

Horse riders should also wear boots or shoes with hard soles and heels. Some have protective toe-caps. Plimsolls, gum boots or trainers are dangerous for riding and should not be worn.

When boots or shoes need repair, through soling is advisable as half-soles can catch in the stirrup irons.

Soft footwear is not acceptable for the BHS Riding and Road Safety Test.

Whip and spurs

It is advisable to carry a whip when riding on the road to act as a back-up to the rider's right leg aid.

Riders with controlled lower leg positions may wish to wear spurs when riding on the roads. These should be short-shanked and properly positioned on the boots.

HAT
Riding gloves – light coloured.
Long-soled boots.
Whip.
Tack – in good condition.
Horse correctly shod.
BE SEEN TO BE SAFE

Riding after dark, at dusk or in inclement/dull weather

▌ Highway Code: Rule 219 – If you have to ride at night, wear reflective clothing and make sure your horse has reflective bands on its legs above the fetlock joints. Carry lights which show white to the front and red to the rear.

This should be avoided where possible by forward planning. If inevitable, reflective clothing should be worn, preferably by both horse and rider to ensure maximum visibility to other road users.

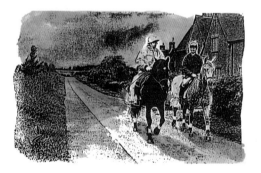

Wearing reflective tabards and leg bands.

It is important to understand the difference between fluorescent and reflective material. Fluorescent materials show up in daylight but have no special qualities at night. Reflective materials return (reflect) a light source either in daylight or darkness. Reflective bands at the fetlock joints are effective and cheap.

A safety lamp should be fitted to the off-side stirrup, showing white to the front, red to the rear.

When leading a horse on foot, the person leading should carry a light in his outside hand, showing white to the front and red to the rear and wear reflective clothing.

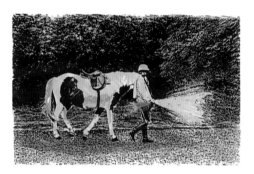

Leading on foot at night.

When in a group, the leading and shepherding off-side riders should wear lights showing white to the front, red to the rear and wear reflective clothing.

Where practicable, light-coloured horses should be placed on the outside.

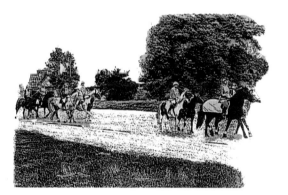

Large riding groups.

REFLECT – INFORM
BE SEEN TO BE SAFE

Reflective material set in yellow gives very good visibility.

An 'L' is recognised by road users as: 'TREAT THE WEARER WITH CAUTION'

TO BE SEEN TO BE SAFE, wear fluorescent and reflective items whenever riding on the public highway.

A selection of road safety clothing and equipment is available from the British Horse Society Marketing Department, British Equestrian Centre, Stoneleigh Park, Kenilworth, Warwickshire, CV8 2LR.

2. THE HIGHWAY CODE

Have you a copy of the current Highway Code? Ask yourself: 'When did I last read it?'

Statutory rules affecting riders

By law:

You **MUST NOT** deliberately ride, lead or drive your horse:

• on a footpath by the side of any road made or set apart for the use of pedestrians (England and Wales);

• on a footway, footpath or cycle track unless there is a right to do so (Scotland).

Children under fourteen **MUST** wear a properly secured approved safety helmet.

Stopping distances

It is important for all riders to be aware of the amount of space needed by a vehicle to stop when travelling at speeds.

REMEMBER:

LORRIES NEED MUCH MORE DISTANCE TO STOP

BE AWARE:

AIR-BRAKES ON HEAVY VEHICLES MAY BLOW OFF AT ANY TIME – THIS IS BEYOND THE DRIVER'S CONTROL

Illustrations for this chapter are taken from the Highway Code © Crown copyright

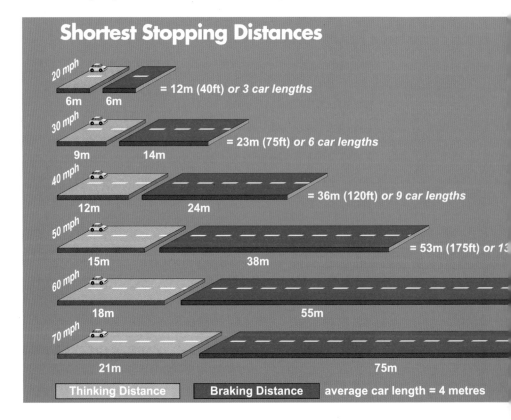

Shortest Stopping Distances

20 mph
6m 6m
= 12m (40ft) *or 3 car lengths*

30 mph
9m 14m
= 23m (75ft) *or 6 car lengths*

40 mph
12m 24m
= 36m (120ft) *or 9 car lengths*

50 mph
15m 38m
= 53m (175ft) *or 13*

60 mph
18m 55m

70 mph
21m 75m

Thinking Distance   Braking Distance   average car length = 4 metres

Traffic light signals

RED means 'Stop'. Wait behind the stop line on the carriageway.

RED AND AMBER also means 'Stop'. Prepare to move off but do not pass through or start until GREEN shows.

GREEN means you may go on if the way is clear. Take special care if you intend to turn left or right and give way to pedestrians who are crossing.

AMBER means 'Stop' at the stop line. You may go on only if the AMBER appears after you have crossed the stop line.

A GREEN ARROW → may be provided in addition to the full green signal if movement in a certain direction is allowed before or after the full green phase. If the way is clear you may go but only in the direction shown by the arrow. You may do this whatever other lights may be showing.

Flashing red lights

At level crossings, lifting bridges, airfields, fire stations etc.

Alternately flashing red lights mean YOU MUST STOP.

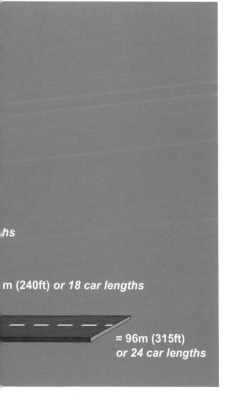

hs

m (240ft) or 18 car lengths

= 96m (315ft)
or 24 car lengths

Road markings across the carriageway

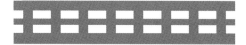

Give way to traffic on major road.

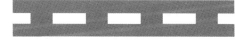

Give way to traffic from the right in roundabout.

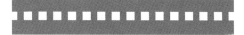

Give way to traffic from right at mini-roundabout.

Stop line at 'STOP' sign.

Stop line at signals or police control.

Signals by authorised persons

STOP | **BECKONING TRAFFIC ON**

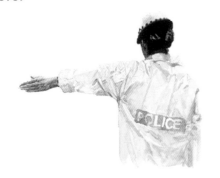

Traffic approaching from behind.

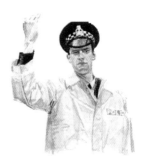

Beckoning on traffic from the front.

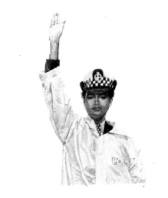

Traffic approaching from the front.

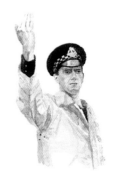

Beckoning on traffic from the side.

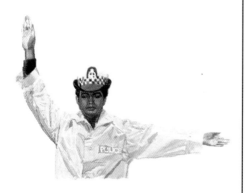

Traffic approaching from both front and behind.

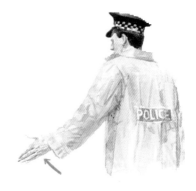

Beckoning on traffic from behind.

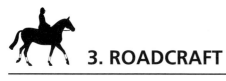
Courtesy

Show courtesy and consideration to all other road users. Take particular care when passing pedestrians, who may be frightened of horses. A friendly greeting from the rider may reassure them. Always thank anyone who slows down or shows any consideration.

A smile and a 'thank you' are usually sufficient to acknowledge considerate drivers. It is unnecessary continually to take the hand from the reins when thanking drivers; both hands on the reins spell better control.

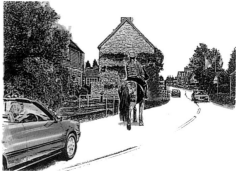

Two vehicles approach from opposite directions with the rider in the middle.

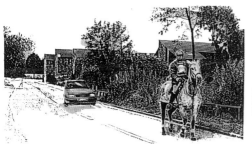

Car approaches rider.

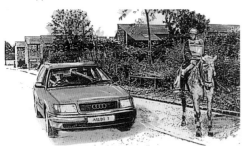

Rider turns to thank driver for slowing down

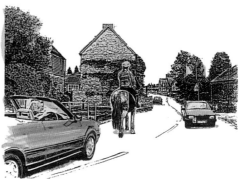

Car waits behind rider.

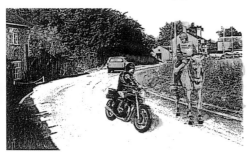

Remember to thank other users of roads and bridleways who give you right of way or show consideration to you.

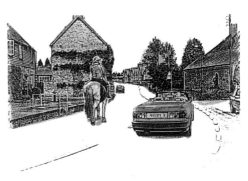

Car overtakes rider. Rider thanks car driver.

Practise good communication with other road users. Your courtesy will be remembered and may benefit other riders.

THE COURTESY CODE
ALWAYS be considerate and help other road users.
ALWAYS acknowledge the courtesy of other road users.
ALWAYS request permission from riders or pedestrians in front of you before passing them on roads or bridleways.
ALWAYS pass other riders or pedestrians at a walk on bridleways or narrow paths.

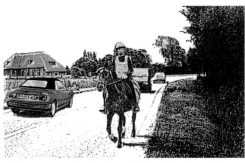

Ride on the left and keep both hands on the reins.

Road awareness

BE AWARE, STAY ALIVE

LOOK, LISTEN AND THINK AHEAD at all times.

> Highway Code: Rule 7c – Look all round for traffic and listen. Traffic could come from any direction, so look along every road. Listen also because you can sometimes hear traffic before you see it.

Be alert for possible hazards, particularly from behind. Look behind regularly to observe the changing road situation.

Bends and corners – be aware of traffic in front and from behind.

On left-hand bends and turns, check over left shoulder for any cyclist or pedestrian on your near side.

AVOID unnecessary or difficult hazards if you can. If trouble looks likely, make a detour to avoid it if at all possible.

AVOID upsetting your horse in traffic.

THE PUBLIC HIGHWAY IS NO PLACE TO TEACH HORSES DISCIPLINE.

Road positioning

Ride on the left of the road. Ride straight and prevent the horse from moving sideways or swinging his quarters into the traffic (by clear use of your leg aids).

Reins must be at the correct length to control the horse.

> Highway Code: Rule 224 – KEEP BOTH HANDS ON THE REINS, unless you are signalling...

OBSERVATION – your position is important, especially at junctions, to give you full and clear visibility of traffic approaching from any direction.

To look behind, turn from the waist, keeping both hands on the reins. LOOK for traffic.

REMEMBER THE ROUTINE:
* OBSERVE
* SIGNAL – clearly and precisely
* OBSERVE
* MANOEUVRE
DON'T DITHER, BE DECISIVE

ALWAYS check the road behind and in front, and where necessary, to the sides. Make sure it is SAFE for you to move.

LOOK BEHIND AND AROUND
SEE TO KEEP SAFE

Riders' signals

> Highway Code: Rule 81 (Motorists) – Look out for horse riders' signals and be aware that they may not move to the centre of the road prior to turning right. Riders of horses and ponies are often children – so take extra care.

> Highway Code: Rule 220 – Before moving off or turning, look behind you to make sure it is safe and then give a clear arm signal...

Before making *any* signal: look, listen and observe.

Take effective observation and respond accordingly.

When it is safe to do so, signal in the direction

you wish to go. Give a last 'life-saver' look. Carry out the manoeuvre.

All signals must be clear and decisive.

Hold your signal for approximately 3 seconds (say, 'one thousand and one, one thousand and two, one thousand and three') to allow sufficient time for other road users to understand your intentions.

NEVER signal with the whip in your hand. To transfer the whip to the left hand, the left thumb is raised, the whip is pushed under that thumb which is then lowered. The right hand is then free to make the signal.

Giving a signal warns other road users of your intentions and is not a guarantee of safety. Other road users may not act responsibly.

Signals for left and right turns

For left and right turns, the arm should be fully extended from the shoulder, hand flat, palm facing the front with the fingers closed.

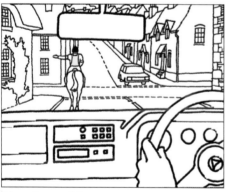

'I intend to turn left.'

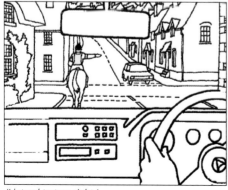

'I intend to turn right.'

Other useful signals

The following signals may be useful in certain circumstances. (Highway Code, Rule 81.) They are requests to other road users.

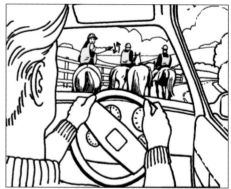

'Driver, please slow down.'

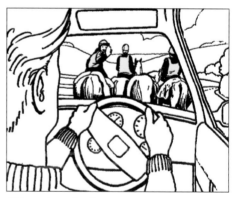

'Driver, please stop.'

> ALWAYS EXPECT THE UNEXPECTED

Horses are unpredictable and need to be given room. Riders should endeavour to influence other road users, not just inform them of their proposed actions. Establish eye contact with other road users.

All riders are vulnerable road users.

An informed driver is usually a more patient driver.

> REMEMBER:
> NEVER move unless it is safe.
> NEVER take a chance – give a 'life-saver' look.
> BE ROAD AWARE – STAY ALIVE.

Positioning at road junctions

> Highway Code: Rule 7f – Keep looking and listening for traffic on approach and if waiting to cross. When you have started to cross, keep looking and listening in case there is any traffic you did not see – or in case other traffic suddenly appears.

ALWAYS check roads to the right and left **as you are crossing**.

Horse riders are vulnerable road users. At all junctions riders should keep to the left, near the kerb or verge. This will avoid riders being sandwiched by other traffic. (If turning left, keep to the left and turn left.)

If you have to wait, reassure your horse, do not fidget him. Keep assessing the traffic situation.

Always keep your horse under control. NEVER allow him to anticipate the move-off.

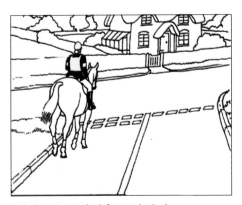

Rider keeping to the left near the kerb.

BE AWARE OF THE TRAFFIC SITUATION
BE ROAD AWARE – STAY ALIVE

T-junctions

Left turns

> Highway Code: Rule 121 – ... watch out for traffic coming up on your left before you make the turn. When turning, keep as close to the left as it is safe so to do.

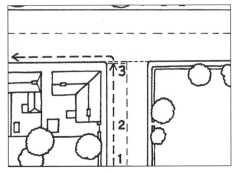

Left turn – minor to major.

1. OBSERVE THE TRAFFIC SITUATION THOROUGHLY.

2. Signal clearly and precisely. Retake the reins. Be prepared to halt for traffic on major road.

3. If necessary to halt, listen. Check traffic situation. Signal clearly. Retake the reins before moving off. 'Life-saver' look over right shoulder; check over left shoulder for cyclists. When safe, proceed, glance right then look in the direction you are travelling.

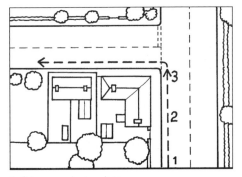

Left turn – major to minor.

1. OBSERVE THE TRAFFIC SITUATION THOROUGHLY.

2. Signal clearly and precisely. Retake the reins.

3. 'Life-saver' look over right shoulder. Check for cyclists over left shoulder. Turn left, keeping as near to the kerb as is safe.

Right turns

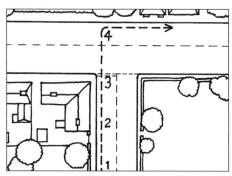

Right turn – minor to major.

1. OBSERVE THE TRAFFIC SITUATION THOROUGHLY.

2. Be prepared to halt (give way).

3. If necessary to halt, listen. Carefully check traffic situation. Signal clearly. Retake the reins. 'Life-saver' look over right shoulder.

4. When clear, walk on briskly, straight across to your new route.

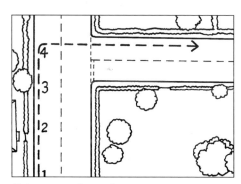

Right turn – major to minor.

1 OBSERVE THE TRAFFIC SITUATION THOROUGHLY.

2. When safe, signal right clearly and precisely. Retake the reins.

3. Carefully check for traffic. If safe, prepare to make a turn opposite your new route, taking the shortest line (4) across the major road.

*If traffic appears on the major road, halt at 4 and continue when safe. If this is dangerous, continue along the major road until it is safe to cross, and return to turn left into the minor road.

Flared junctions

When turning right or left, continue as near as possible along the line of the kerb or verge as if it were a straight junction and position at right-angles to the give-way/stop line.

See and be seen.

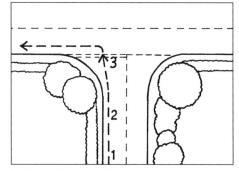

Left turn at flared junction.

1. OBSERVE THE TRAFFIC SITUATION THOROUGHLY.

2. Signal clearly and precisely. Retake the reins. Be prepared to halt.

3. If necessary to halt, listen. Carefully check traffic situation. Signal clearly. Retake the reins before moving off. 'Life-saver' look over right shoulder; check over left shoulder for cyclists. When safe, proceed, looking to the right as you are turning left, then look in direction you are travelling.

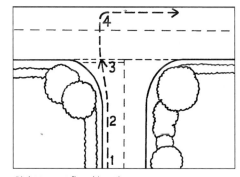

Right turn at flared junction.

1. OBSERVE THE TRAFFIC SITUATION THOROUGHLY.

2. Be prepared to halt.

3. If necessary to halt, listen. Carefully check traffic situation. Signal clearly. Retake the reins. Remember the 'life-saver' look over right shoulder.

4. When clear, walk on briskly, straight across to your new route.

Cross-roads

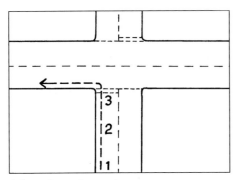

Left turn from minor road.

1. OBSERVE THE TRAFFIC SITUATION THOROUGHLY.

2. Signal clearly and precisely. Retake the reins. Be prepared to halt and give way.

3. At halt listen. Carefully check traffic situation. Check road opposite for traffic emerging. Signal clearly. Retake the reins before moving off. 'Life-saver' look over right shoulder, check over left shoulder for cyclists. When safe, proceed, glancing to the right as you are turning left then look in the direction you are travelling.

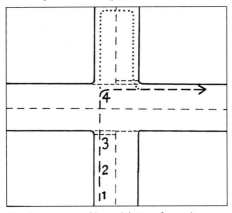

Crossing over or making a right turn from minor road.

1. OBSERVE THE TRAFFIC SITUATION THOROUGHLY.

2. Be prepared to halt.

3. At halt listen. Carefully check traffic situation. Signal clearly if turning. Retake the reins. Remember the 'life-saver' look over right shoulder. When safe, walk briskly, straight across the major road.

4. Position for right turn. However, if road situation dictates, follow dotted route.

Remember: Never fidget your horse. When turning from the major road, follow the procedure as at T-junctions, but OBSERVE CAREFULLY all road conditions.

Traffic lights – These may have filter lanes.

OBSERVE TRAFFIC SITUATION and TRAFFIC LIGHTS.

BEWARE AMBER GAMBLERS

At all times:

Be prepared to halt at traffic lights.

When lights are red or amber, look behind and halt.

KEEP CHECKING THE LIGHTS.

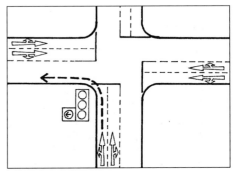

Turning left at traffic lights

When lights are red and amber – look behind, clearly signal your intended direction, and retake the reins before moving off.

When lights are green – check road is clear.

Walk on briskly when it is safe to proceed. Check over left shoulder for cyclists.

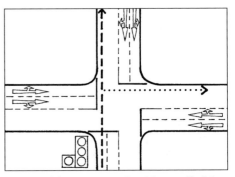

Going straight across or turning right at traffic lights.

When lights are red and amber – check all around that it is safe to proceed. Remember the 'life-saver' look.

When lights turn to green – Walk briskly across, checking to the right and left as you go and the road ahead…

Check that the road is safe before making a right turn, having signalled clearly.

Look behind after completing the turn.

When lights are red *and* amber, LOOK BEHIND, TO THE RIGHT AND LEFT and be ready to proceed.

OBSERVE THE TRAFFIC SITUATION THOROUGHLY AT ALL TIMES.

REMEMBER THE 'LIFE-SAVER' LOOKS.

REMEMBER THE CORRECT PROCEDURE – AT ALL JUNCTIONS.

BE READY TO MOVE OFF IMMEDIATELY IF SAFE TO DO SO, WHEN GREEN LIGHT SHOWS.

Roundabouts

Highway Code: Rule 126 (Motorists) – ... cyclists and horse riders will often keep to the left on the roundabout; they may also indicate right to show they are continuing around the roundabout.

Highway Code: Rule 223 – Avoid roundabouts wherever possible. If you have to use them, keep to the left and watch out for vehicles crossing your path to leave or join the roundabout. Signal right when riding across exits to show you are not leaving. Signal left just before you leave the roundabout.

Roundabouts should be avoided where possible, but if you cannot avoid them, keep to the near side.

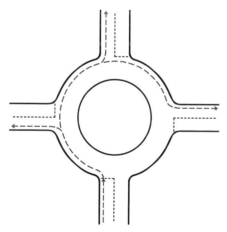

How to tackle a roundabout.

It may not be necessary to signal on the approach to a roundabout, especially when negotiating a major roundabout.

On approach – look behind, then look all around the roundabout, stop if necessary.

To exit – look behind. Signal left, retake reins.

Look behind over right shoulder, then left shoulder. Turn left.

Stationary vehicles

Keep to the left. Look behind in good time. Check for oncoming traffic. Be prepared to hold back for approaching traffic. If safe, signal right, retake the the reins before passing stationary vehicles.

Give a 'life-saver' look behind before moving out round the vehicle. Allow sufficient clearance.

Check on the inside for sudden movement and/or noise from the vehicle.

Where practicable, give such vehicles verbal warning of your presence.

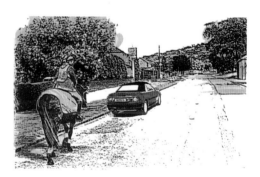

1. Rider looks behind when approaching stationary vehicle.

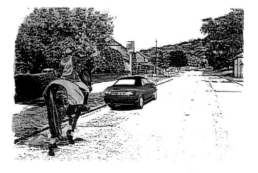

2. Road ahead clear, rider signals.

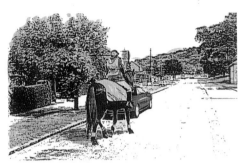

3. Rider takes back reins.

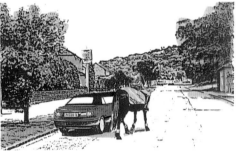

4. Rider starts to overtake vehicle, checking that road is clear.

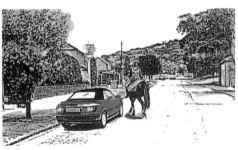

5. Rider overtakes.

If the road is not clear, wait behind vehicle at a sufficient distance to avoid a sharp turn when able to proceed. If you wait too far from the stationary vehicle, you will encourage other vehicles to squeeze between you and the stationary vehicle.

Dangerous/noisy/frightening hazards

(These include road drills, compressors, hedge cutters etc.)

Halt a sufficient distance away.

Reassure your horse.

Try to catch the operator's attention.

Acknowledge any consideration shown.

Do not continue if traffic is approaching.

If your horse will not go forward and you are in company, ask for a lead from another horse.

If you are by yourself, take an alternative route if possible.

If you can foresee a dangerous or frightening hazard, take an alternative route before you arrive at the hazard.

Treat **road works** as a stationary vehicle and follow above procedure unless horse shows resistance to passing.

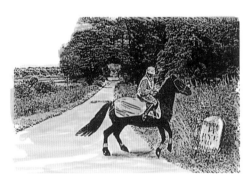

Dangerous: Rider has used his left rein as horse begins to shy. Horse therefore thinks rider wants him to go up to the unfamiliar object, and shies even more, with his hindquarters going out into the road and his right shoulder escaping.

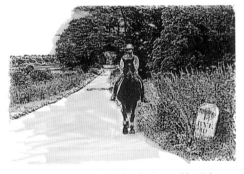

Safer: Rider has used right leg (supported by right rein) to bend horse away from the unfamiliar object before he starts to shy. Right rein controls horse's right shoulder and rider's right leg controls the hindquarters and keeps him straight. Left leg keeps him moving forward and on the bit.

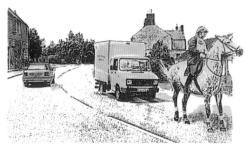

Dangerous: Rider has allowed horse to see lorry with his left eye. He keeps his eye on the frightening lorry and his hindquarters swing out into its path.

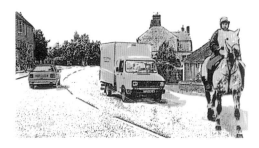

Safer: Rider uses right leg (supported by right rein) to make sure that horse sees lorry with his right eye. Rider's right leg pushes horse's hindquarters to the side of the road away from the lorry, and left leg keeps horse on the bit and going forward.

Railway bridges

OBSERVE TRAFFIC SITUATION.

Halt in good time if necessary.

Listen for oncoming trains.

Never ride over or under a bridge if a train is approaching.

Bridges and underpasses

Bridges and underpasses provided to cross trunk roads and motorways are helpful to riders but can present hazards. Headroom in underpasses can be low – dismount and lead through if necessary. Some parapets provided on bridges are not high enough. If in doubt, dismount and lead across.

When negotiating bridges and underpasses, wait for pedestrians to cross first.

Grass verges and footpaths

> Highway Code: Rule 222 – You **MUST NOT** take a horse on to a footpath, pavement or cycle track. Use a bridlepath where possible.

If it is practicable, ride on verges, unless the local council has a bye-law forbidding this.

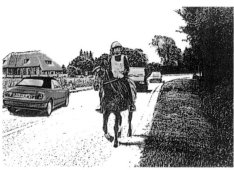

Verge too narrow.

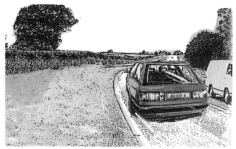

Verge wide enough.

It is hazardous and foolish to canter on verges

Give way to any pedestrian using a pedestrian crossing.

Dismounting, leading and remounting

> Highway Code: Rule 220 – … When riding, keep to the left. If you are leading a horse, keep it to your left…

Dismount only if it is essential to do so. The safest place is usually on the horse's back.

If dismounting is inevitable, it should be done quickly, safely and efficiently, with the rider in control.

It is customary to dismount on the near side.

There are circumstances when dismounting and/or remounting on the off-side is helpful, but this will require practice.

Whichever side you intend to remount, near or off, that stirrup should be crossed over first. The horse should be 'pointing' in the direction of the traffic flow.

Leading horses when dismounted

Gloves should always be worn by the leader. **The led horse must always wear a bridle. Lead on the left of the road.**

The leader should be positioned at the horse's head, between the horse and the traffic.

When leading a horse wearing a running martingale, leave the reins on his neck, hold them in the left hand approximately 10cm (4 inches) behind the bit. A whip should be held in the right hand to help control the horse's quarters.

When leading horses on foot, along the road, **the horse must always wear a bridle.**

Leading when mounted

If you lead when mounted, ride on the left-hand side of the road with the led horse on your left side, away from the traffic.

When a horse is led from another, the led horse should wear a bridle with the reins passed through the bit to the right side. If the led horse is wearing a running martingale, it should be securely tied up and free of the reins.

Riding in pairs or groups

> Highway Code: Rule 221 – Never ride more than two abreast. Ride in single file where circumstances dictate.

Groups of riders should not exceed eight.

Riders should proceed in pairs, with a minimum of 1.3m (4ft), nose to tail, between horses.

With large groups of riders, e.g. a sponsored ride, groups should be divided, leaving a minimum of 30m (100ft) between groups.

Before the group sets out, the procedure for moving into single file from double file and back to single file should be established and fully understood by all group members.

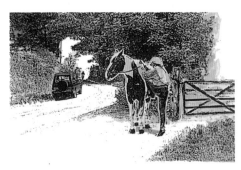

Making use of a gateway.

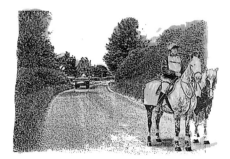

Leading with a bridle.

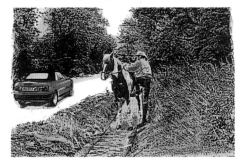

A fold in the ground or verge can be useful.

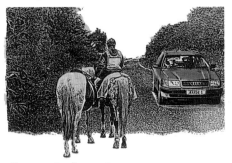

Keep over to allow car to pass.

A method of communication should be established in case of difficulties; the plan of the ride and the expected time of return should be given to a responsible member of staff at the home base before the ride leaves.

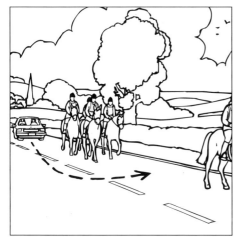

Car approaches group of eight riders. Riders have left a gap so that car may overtake first group. Car overtakes first group of riders.

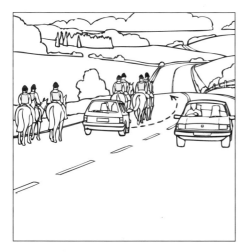

Car stays tucked in between groups while oncoming vehicle passes in other lane. When road is clear, car overtakes leading group of riders.

Although obstruction of other road users should be avoided, alert, defensive riding should be practised to avoid rash overtaking by other road users.

Fluorescent and reflective tabards are important visibility aids for all riders.

The ride leader should be mature and safety conscious, of a minimum age of sixteen years, and fully understand the applicable legal and insurance responsibilities before taking groups of riders and horses onto the public highway.

There should be an able 'shepherd' at the rear of the group.

Arm signals and traffic appreciation should be made by the leader and shepherd respectively. They should be in full control of the group, and have a pre-agreed method of communication with each other.

Young and inexperienced horses and riders should be on the inside of older, experienced horses and riders.

The pace set by the group leader should be one that all members can safely and comfortably maintain.

Courtesy is imperative when other road users have been delayed by the group.

Take single file as circumstances dictate.

Groups of riders from riding schools

It may be more practicable for the ride to remain closed up. If school animals are separated, the herd instinct may assert itself, which could become hazardous to other road users.

Road junctions should be crossed as a controlled group, monitored by the person in charge.

Defensive riding

ALL RIDERS ARE PART OF THE TRAFFIC.

On occasions it may be necessary, sensible and safe to take up the amount of road normally used by a motor vehicle.

For example:

(a) Take up a more visible position on the road, rather than riding too close to the edge. Vehicles should then slow down to overtake.

(b) Where conditions permit, two or more riders may ride in pairs.

In both examples, great care should be taken not to obstruct traffic unduly, except when safety so dictates.

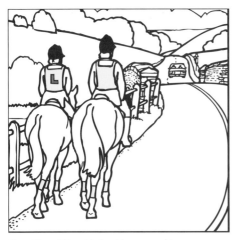

Two riders riding side by side approaching a narrow bridge. They see a car coming towards them.

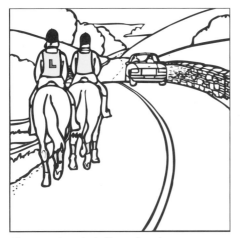

They move into single file to allow the car to pass.

When safe or if necessary, either pull into the side of the road or move into single file to allow traffic to overtake.

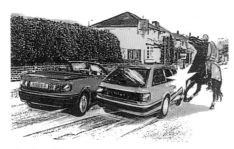

Classic accident.

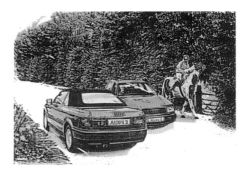

Classic accident.

The above illustration is a situation that would have justified a rider requesting the driver approaching from behind either to slow down or stop. See illustrations on page 17; ...'riders should endeavour to influence other road users'.

BE READY TO MOVE OUT OF THE WAY QUICKLY if necessary. BE ALERT.

BEWARE BLIND CORNERS/ROAD NARROWING.

THANK CONSIDERATE DRIVERS.

Dangerous road conditions

Worn, shiny patches on roads are dangerous.

Plastic paint, as used for white lines and zebra crossings, is slippery.

Do not trot round corners – most are slippery.

BEWARE!

Proprietary anti-slip studs, nails and horseshoes can provide additional grip.

Snow and ice

When snow or ice is about, road conditions become more dangerous.

If exercising MUST take place, keep your horse at a walk and allow him to take his time.

Ride as near to the kerb, gutter or edge of the road as is safe.

Grit or dirt will provide a better footing.

Keep a rein contact with the horse at all times.

It is advisable to remove your feet from the stirrup irons and cross the irons over the horse's neck.

If the horse slips and falls – DON'T PANIC.

Keep calm, allow the horse to regain his footing in his own time. Check the horse for injury.

Move off the icy road before remounting.

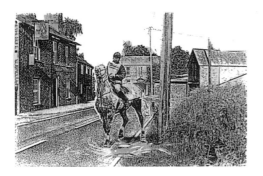

When riding in snow, smear grease thickly on the frogs and soles of the horse's four feet, to help prevent snow 'balling' in the hoof. Carry a folding hoof-pick for removal of snow.

Leading a horse on foot on an icy road

Allow the horse to go at his own pace.

Concentrate on your own footing.

Fog and mist

If caught in fog or mist – take the same precautions as when riding at dusk or dark.

BE PREPARED.

All these conditions should be avoided wherever possible. Give your horse a day off, rather than become another accident statistic.

Horse and equipment

The horse must be used to carrying a side-saddle, and must answer to the rigid whip.

The saddle must be in good condition and the tree must be sound. Special attention must be paid to the fixed pommel and the leaping head.

Buckles, bends and stitching must be in good repair.

The fit at the wither, shoulder and spine is important, with no pinching.

The seat should be level front to back. Packing on the near-side rear-panel must be greater than that on the off-side, *to allow the seat to sit level from side to side when the rider is in position.*

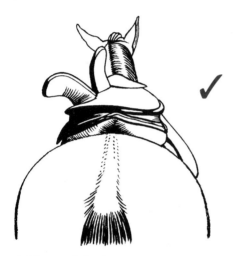

Saddle correctly fitted.

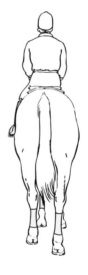

Rider sitting square, seat level from side to side.

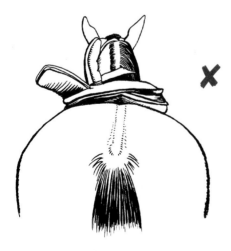

Saddle tilting left.

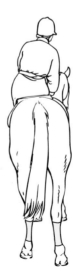

Insufficient packing on both sides, especially near side.

Ideally the girth should be made of leather, and either plain or three-fold. It should be smooth, with a central keeper to accommodate a full-length balance strap and flap strap. The balance strap must be used.

Stirrup attachment – the safety fittings on the saddle and at the top of the stirrup leather must be in accord with the make of saddle.

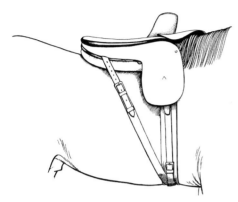

Position of balance strap in relation to girth.

The stirrup iron must be 12mm (½ inch) wider than the rider's boot. It should be in good condition and preferably of stainless-steel. If a roller bar is fitted to the saddle, the stirrup iron must be a safety-release type.

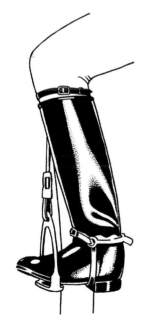

Leather guard must cover billet hook. Note correctly fitted spur.

Rider

A side-saddle habit need not be worn.

The rider's hat must conform to BS EN 1384 (97) or PAS 015 (94).

A whip or rigid cane must be carried, a maximum length of 1m (39 inches), for use as a right leg aid.

A spur or spur-band may be worn by adult riders.

Note: Gloves should be light coloured to aid clarity of signals.

For advice on fit and condition of side-saddles, contact the local SSA Area Chairman or an instructor from the SSA Panel. (In case of difficulties, contact Mrs M. James, SSA Hon. Secretary, Highbury House, 19 High Street, Welford, Northampton, NN6 7HT. Tel: 01858 575300.)

Side-saddle riders must be competent riding sideways, and be able to control their horse in walk, trot and canter. They must understand and be able to use the rigid whip to the correct effect.

To maintain control of the horse's quarters and ensure clear visibility over the right shoulder, side-saddle riders can approach hazards and junctions in a shallow 'shoulder fore' to the right.

There are no special concessions for side-saddle riders, in either control of the horse or safety.

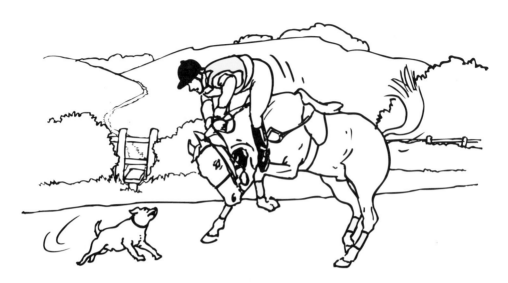

Although the highway provides a very hostile environment for horse and rider, only the very few will be able to avoid it during the course of a ride. In order to minimise the hazards encountered alertness, anticipation, conspicuity and a defensive approach will stand one in good stead. Remember it is no place for the inexperienced horse or rider. Unfortunately, circumstances may be outside one's control and even competent riders may be thrown from a startled horse with consequent injury. It would be natural to panic in such a situation, but this can be controlled if one has learned a basic order of actions to be taken. The aim will be to prevent further harm.

Immediately secure the scene of the accident

1. Send a group member to warn oncoming traffic (in both directions if possible) to slow down or stop.

2. If a horse or pony is loose, attempt to have it caught and led to rejoin the others.

3. Ask someone to summon the **EMERGENCY SERVICES** – usually police and ambulance. Tell them it will be necessary to describe the exact location. A veterinary surgeon may also be needed.

See Highway Code: Rule 153.

When carrying out these immediate steps and going to help the fallen rider, remember your own safety and that of the others is of paramount importance. Do not take unnecessary risks.

Start the ABC of Emergency Aid

A
APPROACH:

Ensure that it is safe to approach the fallen rider because a second accident now may make matters much worse.

ASSESS:

How bad is the injury?

If the rider is conscious, ask if there is pain anywhere.

If so, tell the rider to lie still and not to move if possible. Reassure by confirming that skilled help has been sent for and by listening to what the rider has to say.

A rider who complains of pain in the neck or back must not sit up or stand up until it has confidently been established by skilled examination that an injury cannot be made any worse.

ASSISTANCE:

Call for it if a rider is distressed or not moving.

AIRWAY:

If the rider has not responded to the questions 'Can you hear me?', 'Are you alright?' or a gentle tap or shake on the shoulder, **then the most urgent priority is the Airway. Seconds count.**

A STANDS FOR
AIRWAY AND
ATTENTION
TO IT **ALWAYS**

The airway is the passage through the nose and mouth by which air containing oxygen reaches the lungs. It can be obstructed by the tongue resting at the back of the throat (or uncommonly by debris if the fall has been on to the face) if the rider is unconscious.

The airway is cleared of obstruction from the tongue by lifting the chin upwards and forwards at the same time as an assistant prevents the head and neck from movement.

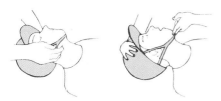

The chin is lifted by two fingertips placed under the point of the chin with gentle pressure applied to the rider's forehead with the other hand. The hat is not removed to do this although it may be necessary carefully to undo the chinstrap.

Remember the tongue is attached to the lower jaw (mandible) and will be lifted away from the back of the throat as the chin is moved. Obviously it will be necessary to maintain the chin in the correct position or the tongue will fall back again.

Air must reach the lungs, even when a serious neck injury is suspected, and opening the airway is a most urgent and vital step.

If loose dentures (well fitting ones must be left in place) or foreign matter are seen to be causing an obstruction they must be cautiously removed. At all costs remember that pushing anything further down the throat or causing gagging must be avoided.

Tight clothing around the neck may have to be loosened.

Once the airway is clear the next step is to check the rider is breathing.

B
STANDS FOR **BREATHING**
LOOK, LISTEN AND FEEL FOR 5 SECONDS

The ear placed close to the rider's mouth and nose may hear the sound of normal breathing (or obstructed breathing if the airway has not been adequately opened), breath may be felt on the cheek and the chest seen to rise and fall whilst looking towards the rider's feet.

If, despite an open airway, the rider cannot be seen, felt or heard to be breathing, then the carotid pulse in the neck must be checked. Remember to feel for 5 seconds if it is thought to be absent. If it cannot be felt then the technique of C.P.R. (Cardio-Pulmonary Resuscitation) must be used (see below).

Fortunately, it is very unlikely that the rider's heart has stopped beating and the next step is to provide mouth-to-mouth ventilation.

Ten breaths (10) are given before checking the carotid pulse again.

It may be necessary to log-roll the rider into the face-up position (controlling the head and neck) in order to do this.

After taking a full breath in, and pinching the rider's nostrils closed with the thumb and finger of the hand that is not supporting the chin, the lips of the rescuer are placed around the slightly open mouth of the rider. A steady blow of air is given over about 2 seconds, enough to see the chest rise. In order to allow the rider's breath to escape and the lungs to deflate, the rescuer's mouth is then removed. This ventilation is repeated 10 times before another check on the carotid pulse. It must be continued until such time as the rider can breathe again or the medical team can take over the task.

C
C STANDS FOR **CIRCULATION**

In the rare event of the carotid pulse not being felt it will be necessary to combine chest compressions with mouth-to-mouth ventilation. The single rescuer will provide 2 breaths alternating with 15 compressions (two rescuers will combine 1 breath with 5 compressions).

It is the duty of all competent people to be able to provide such skills, which are most often required for victims of a heart attack sustaining a cardiac arrest. The purchase of the First Aid Manual of The British Red Cross Society, St Andrew's Ambulance Association and St John Ambulance from a bookshop will illustrate these techniques. The necessary training may be obtained by application to local branches of these organisations.

Remember, revision will be necessary to maintain these skills.

If the rider is conscious

It is much more likely that injury will have damaged the circulatory system and bleeding will have occurred.

In order to stop bleeding, a careful search must be made for the source and then pressure applied to the wound.

This may have to be with thumb or fingers, but a clean pad between them and the wound is preferable. Firm pressure is maintained.

Remember, a simple nose bleed requires pressure on the soft part of the nose and not on the bony bridge of the nose. The rider may be able to do this whilst breathing through the mouth.

Severe bleeding (which may be internal) can lead to a state of shock. It is important, if this is a possibility, to disturb the rider as little as possible and to keep the rider lying down.

Protection from the elements must be considered and provided.

If the rider is unconscious

If breathing normally, a decision will have to be made to log-roll the rider onto the side. The reason for this is that there is the deadly hazard of inhaling into the lungs fluid from the mouth, vomit or the contents that seep up unseen from the stomach. If the airway is adjusted properly, it will also prevent the tongue from falling back to cause an obstruction.

In order to log-roll safely, without harm to the rider, it will be necessary to turn the rider's head, neck and back as one unit. This will require the help of at least three or four others. The most experienced helper should take control of the head and neck and then orchestrate the timing of the turn.

In practice, it is easier to work on the opposite side of the casualty to your partner.

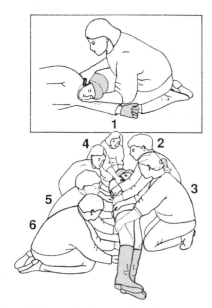

In this illustration the numbered positions depend on the availability of helpers. 2 and 3 are essential, then 4 and 5 with 6 placed either side.

When the log-roll is completed, nos 1, 2 and 3 remain until replaced by trained personnel.

It could just be there is no-one to help if an accident happens in remote circumstances. The unconscious companion can still be turned onto the side by making use of the arm that is nearest to the rescuer. Unlike the recovery position, when the arm is placed at a right-angle to the body and then bent at the elbow, the arm is put above the rider's head as if in the back-stroke position for swimming.

Then, after bending the rider's knee that is furthest away to a right-angle, the rider's head is kept supported by his arm as the rescuer grasps the clothing at the far hip and pulls slowly.

The turn is made towards the rescuer's knees in order to provide the greatest support and control. The airway is checked, re-adjusted if necessary, and then the rider's bent knee is also adjusted to provide the necessary support preventing any further tendency to roll forwards. However, this turn is only used if no help can be obtained.

In summary, once the scene of the accident has been secured, apply the ABC of

immediate care. It must be in the correct sequence for the airway must have the greatest priority if the injured rider is unconscious. Remember, just correctly positioning the rider's chin may be enough not only to restart breathing but also literally to save their life. If the unconscious rider does not need assistance to breathe, and if skilled help is not at hand, the rider will require a log-roll turn into the recovery position using as many helpers as possible.

The airway must be checked and re-checked constantly.

Finally, remember to record all the details of the accident as soon as you reasonably can and to complete the BHS Accident Report (provided at the back of this book).

Insurance – Are you legally liable?

It was stated at the beginning of this Manual that under certain circumstances a rider is likely to be considered liable if his horse or pony causes any harm to other people or their property, and may be liable to pay considerable damages. It is therefore strongly advisable for riders and horse-owners to take out appropriate insurance. Free personal liability insurance is automatically extended to members of the British Horse Society who have Full Adult, Full Junior, Founder or Life Membership and who live in, or are visiting, the United Kingdom or Eire. Note that Associate Members are not covered.

You should also note that personal liability insurance covers **legal** not **moral** liability.

Indemnity – £2,000,000 in respect of any one accident.

Cover – Members should consult the BHS Yearbook for full details of cover. In brief, cover is extended in most foreseeable circumstances for individual members. Block cover for officials at events is also extended to all equestrian activities organised by individual members of the Society or its Committees, by the Pony Club or its Branches, by affiliated riding groups and by affiliated bridlepath groups.

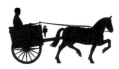
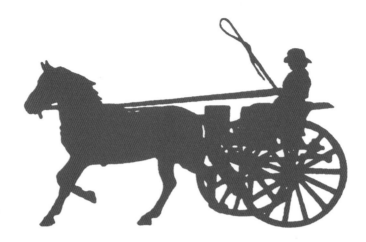

The logo of the British Driving Society.

The Highway Code applies as much to the driven as to the ridden horse or motor vehicle. It must be studied and complied with at all times. The same basic principles also apply to safety.

Before going on the road

Before going on the road not only the harness but also the vehicle's brakes, if any, wheels and shafts should be carefully checked. Should this disclose either wear or damage, the vehicle should be put into good working order before being driven on, or off, the road.

Two-wheeled vehicles must be correctly balanced.

Harness should be checked and all stitching regularly examined for wear.

All leather should be pliant and correctly dressed.

Harness should be comfortably fitted and suitable for both the horse and vehicle.

The breeching should be adjusted to prevent the vehicle running into the horse, and blinkers, if worn, should prevent the horse from seeing to the rear.

Headcollars, if worn, should be fitted correctly.

On the road

In the interests of safety, do not go out on the road with an animal that is young, nervous or traffic-shy. Until he has developed confidence, ride him or lead him on the road only in company with traffic-trained horses, and always try to avoid peak traffic times.

Do not drive on the road until you know that you can control your horse. Response to the driver's voice is particularly important and will help you both to drive a steady unwavering course beside the kerb and ensure that your horse does not shy or deviate from its course when faced with sudden changes such as manhole covers, different road surfaces or white road markings.

Drive an even course near the left hand kerb – a wide gap may tempt a cyclist or motor cyclist to overtake on the near side.

When driving in congested traffic, try to time your speed and stopping distance to allow space around your turn-out.

You are strongly advised to have an active passenger as an assistant, who can alight before blind bends and junctions and walk ahead to check that it is safe to proceed. If there is any doubt as to whether your animal will stand still at a junction where you have to stop, ask your assistant to dismount and hold the animal's head.

At railway bridges stop well back and listen for oncoming trains. Proceed only when you are sure you will not be caught in the vicinity of the bridge when a train is passing above or below, as this may startle the horse.

As horse-drawn vehicles are slower-moving than motorised traffic, take care to prevent a build-up of traffic behind you.

Use unfrequented roads if possible; if not, drive alertly, and be ready to let other road users overtake (when safe to do so), by moving your horse-drawn vehicle to the left of the road.

Always drive holding both reins in the left hand with the right assisting to keep the horse on the chosen course. By holding the reins in the left hand, the right hand is free to carry a whip and make clear hand signals.

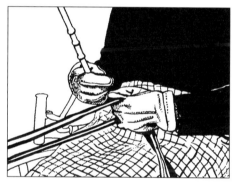

Holding reins properly.

You should know how to make left and right turning signals using the whip in the right hand: when a turn to the right is intended, the whip is held horizontally to the right; a left hand turn is signalled by holding the whip horizontally to the left.

Only use whip signals to following horse-drawn vehicles – motor-vehicle drivers are more likely to understand hand signals.

Slow down and be prepared to stop when ridden ponies or horses are near. Animals unused to seeing horses and ponies being driven often take fright.

When driving the same rule applies as when riding:

BE SEEN TO BE SAFE

Reflectors on driven vehicles are mandatory. They will require front lamps, rear position lamps and rear retro reflectors. Details of these requirements will be found in 'The Road Vehicles Lighting Regulations 1989', available from Her Majesty's Stationery Office.

Wear light or reflective clothing or attach a fluorescent panel to the rear of your vehicle, so that the turn-out is easily seen by approaching vehicles.

Driving in the dusk or in half light is very ill-advised, but if unavoidable, it is essential that driven vehicles now show **'white lights to the front and red to the rear after lighting-up time.'**

7. BRITISH HORSE SOCIETY RIDING AND ROAD SAFETY TEST

The aim

The aim of the test is to give recognition to responsible, courteous and competent riders well versed in roadcraft and road safety as set out within this Manual and the current edition of the Highway Code.

Riding ability – All potential candidates for the BHS Riding and Road Safety Test must be capable of riding independently at walk, trot and canter.

Tack and turn-out inspection – Before the test, a tack and turn-out inspection is held. This is entirely a safety measure carried out to make sure that the horse's tack and the rider's clothing are in a safe and satisfactory condition for riding. It is neither a test nor a 'show' inspection. Hats must be to current British Standards and properly secured. **Cycling helmets are not acceptable unless certified and Kite-marked to current standards.**

The test

The test itself is divided into three parts:

PART 1: THEORY TEST

This is designed to test a rider's knowledge of the Highway Code, the meaning of traffic signs and signals and the generally accepted rules for riding on the highway as set out within this booklet. Questions may be given orally or in the form of a test paper. Ten questions will be asked of each candidate and may be multi-choice, direct or a combination of both. When oral questions are put, each candidate should be seen individually, and asked ten questions, which call for factual answers not opinions. (See sample questions, page 43.)

PART 2: SIMULATED ROAD ROUTE

This is designed to test, in a controlled, safe, simulated road situation, a rider's precautions against - and reactions to - a series of noises and sights which might reasonably be met on the road, and which might make a horse shy. Hazards shall be so placed as to permit candidates to show **trot** between each or any

of them. Road junctions must be included so that candidates may demonstrate control, roadcraft, and their ability to use arm signals. **TROT MUST BE SHOWN.**

PART 3: ROAD TEST ON THE PUBLIC HIGHWAY

This is designed to test riders' roadcraft, road awareness, knowledge and application of the requirements of the Highway Code and of this Manual, in genuine road situations.

As on the Simulated Road Route, the test must be ridden individually. Trot **MUST** be shown by all candidates on the public highway. The stretch of public highway chosen should afford candidates the opportunity to demonstrate their grasp of roadcraft and awareness, together with their riding ability.

Notes for organisers

Administration

1 *Organising the test*. This is the responsibility of the BHS Regional or County Road Safety Representative, who must be contacted to confirm the proposed dates at least one month in advance. Notification should be made at that time if there are side-saddle riders or candidates with special needs.

A Side-Saddle Association 'A' Panel instructor will need to be in attendance at the test, to examine the fit of the saddle and answer any questions the BHS Riding and Road Safety Examiner may have. Side-saddle candidates will benefit from having an experienced person to give them a leg-up.

2 *A Local Authority Road Safety Officer or Police Officer* should be invited to attend by the BHS Road Safety Representative, as their support and expertise is much appreciated.

3 *Application forms, fees, insurance cover.* Application forms must be completed and test fees received from candidates before the test takes place. Insurance cover includes both third party legal liability and personal accident during the test. All fees and a list of names and addresses of successful candidates is to be sent to the Safety Office, Stoneleigh Park, within twenty-four hours.

4 *Nominal roll.* A list of candidates should be prepared and each one allocated a number on arrival for the test. A corresponding supply of numbered fluorescent BHS Road Safety Tabards should be provided.

5 *Briefing stewards.* Arrangements must be made to brief the markers on assessing the performance of candidates. Sufficient time should be allowed for this, on or before the day of the test. (See example marking sheets below.)

6 *Insurance.* The BHS Regional/County Road Safety Representatives and Examiners are covered under the BHS Corporate Public Liability Policy up to £20,000,000. Trainers for BHS Road Safety Tests are covered only when working with the written authority of their Riding and Road Safety Representative.

Simulated road test marking sheet.

Candidate	Date	Examiner	
	Comments		P / B / F
Hazard 1			
Hazard 2			
Hazard 3			
Hazard 4			
Hazard 5			
Hazard 6			
Hazard 7			
Hazard 8			
Hazard 9			
Hazard 10			
Trot			
Dismount, leading & remount			
Control			
Road craft			
Total Pass / fail			

Road test marking sheet.

Candidate's Number	Traffic lights	Being overtaken	Being passed	Overtake stationary car	Move off	Left turn	I-junction	Right turn	Pass or fail

Where such instruction or testing takes place under the auspices of an approved riding school, their third party legal liability insurance cover will, or should, embrace the people employed in this work as far as their negligence may be concerned.

Where the BHS Road Safety Representative for the County is requested by a licensed but not approved riding school to instruct them and their pupils, e.g. on riding and road safety, then the individual instructor is covered under the corporate policy of the BHS, but the individuals employed by the school to carry out instructions are not, unless they are protected under the school's own third party policy.

Side-Saddle Association Panel instructors must be covered by their own insurance.

Candidates over the age of seventy years must take out their own third party legal liability insurance cover.

7 *Police.* It is sensible and polite to inform the local police that a test is taking place. Details of the proposed road route should be made clear.

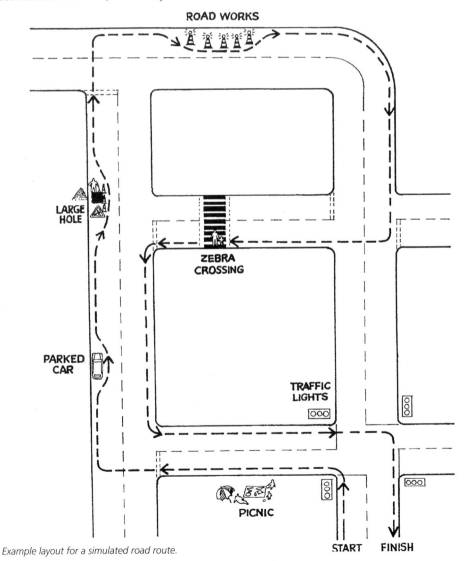

Example layout for a simulated road route.

Personnel

1 *Listed Riding and Road Safety Examiners.* If appropriate, the BHS County Road Safety Representative should inform the Side-Saddle Association so that a listed 'A' Panel Instructor may be invited to attend the test, to examine the fit of the saddle and answer any questions the BHS Riding and Road Safety Examiner may have.

The Examiner on this section must have a writer to take down marks and comments. On the simulated road test it is advisable for the examiner to have a writer.

2 *Stewards.* A sufficient number are required to observe and mark candidates at each point of the road test.

One steward may adjudicate at more than one station depending on how the road test is arranged.

Venue

It is essential that a suitable road route be planned on the public highway. A suitable off-road area is required for the simulated road section. Both these needs must be taken into account when planning a test site.

Once a possible site has been selected, the BHS Regional/County Road Safety Representative should be invited to inspect and approve the proposed public highway and simulated road routes. These will either be approved or alternative routes given.

1 The off-road area should be flat and about 100 x 100m (100 x 100yds).

2 The road route should contain the required hazards and be of such length as to ensure a realistic test with sufficient, but not dangerous, traffic flow. Suggested formats appear below and overleaf.

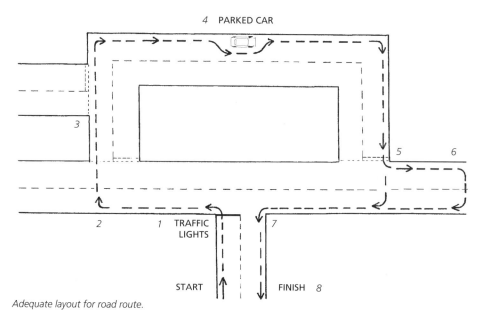

Adequate layout for road route.

START

1. Traffic lights (left turn minor to major)
2. Right turn (major to minor)
3. Approaching and passing road junction
4. Overtaking stationary vehicle
5. Turning right (minor to major)
6. Alternative route
7. Left turn (major to minor)
8. Finish

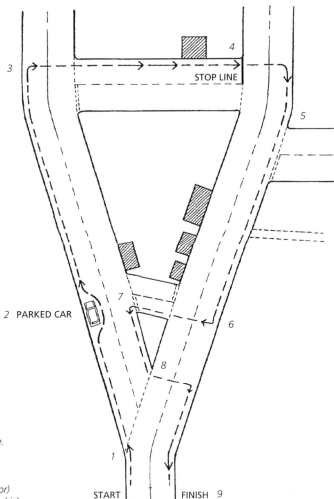

Ideal layout for road route.

START

1. Left turn (major to minor)
2. Overtaking stationary vehicle
3. Right turn (major to minor)
4. Stop at major road (right turn minor to major)
5. Approaching and passing road junction
6. Right turn (major to minor)
7. Left turn (minor to major)
8. Right turn (minor to major)
9. Finish

Candidates should ride the test on their own horse/pony where possible, or on the horse/pony they usually ride.

The same horse/pony may be used for two candidates only.

Equipment and materials

The following items will be required:

- Candidates' numbered fluorescent jackets.

- Pencils and clip-boards.
- Marking sheets for all examiners and stewards.
- Summary sheet.

These may be provided by the BHS County Road Safety Representative.

A diagram of both the simulated and road test routes should be on display for examiners, stewards and candidates.

1 *Theory test*
- A covered area at or adjacent to the test site is ideal.

2 *Simulated road route*
- Traffic lights – miniature or actual size.
- Road signs – miniature or actual size.
- Sawdust, lime, cones, fire hose, tape or white guttering for marking roads and junctions.

The BHS Regional/County Road Safety Representative may be able to provide some of these items.

On the day of the test, the simulated road route may be altered at the discretion of the examiners.

3 *Road route*
- Vehicle as a hazard.
- Cones if necessary.

Organiser's checklist
1. Select date and time of test.
2. Notify Regional Road Safety Representative and Development Officer
3. Enlist stewards.
4. Select venue for approval by BHS County Road Safety Representative.
5. Obtain equipment and materials.

Procedure on test day – BHS County/Regional Road Safety Representative.

All three parts of the test must be taken on the same day.

1 *Marshalling candidates.* Application forms should be collected by the organiser and given to the BHS County Road Safety Representative, together with any test fees not received before the test day. Cheques should be made payable to: British Horse Society Safety Department.

2 *Theory test.* Administer theory paper. The answers should be marked and transferred to the master sheet. Candidates can now collect their horses for the tack, turn-out and hat inspection.

3 *Tack and turn-out inspection of horse and rider.* This is a safety measure carried out to ensure that the horse's tack and the rider's clothing are in a safe and satisfactory condition for riding. It is neither a test nor a 'show' inspection.

4 *Simulated road route.* Candidates move on to this test upon completion of the theory and tack and turn-out sections. **It is a test of the rider**, not the horse. However, if a horse appears unsafe in Part 2, the candidate will not be allowed to attempt Part 3 on that horse. At the BHS Examiner's discretion, a candidate may be allowed to change onto another horse. The candidate must then ride the simulated road test again, to satisfy the examiner on his/her control of the 'new' horse and road safety knowledge.

5 *Public highway.* Candidates proceed to this section upon passing the theory and simulated road route sections.

To be successful, the candidate must satisfy the examiners in the three parts of the test consecutively. A candidate failing in either Part 1 or 2 cannot take Part 3.

Eight of the ten theory questions must be correctly answered.

Candidates on the road section must be examined individually, although there may be more than one candidate on the road at a time.

Candidates must satisfy the examiners in Parts 2 and 3 at a level of 80%. Any manoeuvre which is judged as dangerous to other road users or to the candidate will result in instant failure, e.g. not looking behind before giving a signal, or failing to assess the road situation safely and to the examiners' satisfaction.

6 *Collection of marked sheets.* To expedite final marking, it is helpful to transfer marks already obtained onto the master sheet, e.g. from the theory and simulated sections, and collect from stewards at intervals throughout the test.

7 *Certificates.* These are issued directly to successful candidates by the Safety Office, Stoneleigh Park, where certification is recorded.

8 *Successful candidates.* These will receive a Riding and Road Safety badge. They will be spoken to by all the examiners, and told of their strengths and weaknesses.

9 *Unsuccessful candidates.* These will be tactfully spoken to individually by the examiners, and told of their strong points, together with their weak ones. They will be encouraged to undertake training and another test at the earliest suitable opportunity.

Notes for candidates

1 The minimum age is twelve years. The maximum age is seventy years, unless that person takes out his own insurance. Horses must be four years old or over.

2 Before the test – it is important that candidates are properly prepared for the BHS Riding and Road Safety Test. This preparation should come via the BHS County Road Safety Representative and team of Riding and Road Safety Instructors, enabling a programme of correct training to be given.

3 Required reading/viewing:

- *Ride More Safely.*
- The current *BHS Riding and Road Safety Test Card.*
- The current *BHS Manual of Riding and Roadcraft.*
- The current edition of the *Highway Code*, available from HMSO, the BHS and most bookshops.

Additional reading:

'Horse Sense: Roadcraft for the Rider' – a 20-minute video.

Know your Traffic Signs.

The Pony Club Road Safety Video.

The Highway Code for Children – available from the BHS Bookshop, BEC, Stoneleigh Park, Kenilworth, Warks, CV8 2LR. Prices on application.

The Highway Code Video

Lessons

A minimum of six training sessions are required. More may be needed. Ideally, these should be spread over several weeks to ensure a thorough understanding of the subject. Parents are advised to attend training sessions too, so that they may understand the subject as well.

Suggested guidelines for training sessions

These can be altered or re-organised where necessary, to accommodate potential candidates who need longer to assimilate the necessary knowledge.

For mounted and unmounted training sessions, an assistant is useful. Parents should also attend, if applicable.

At the instructor's discretion, candidates may be taught individually on the road.

When possible, assess candidates' riding ability before road safety training begins. This will be covered in more detail in the Riding and Road Safety Instructor's and Examiner's folder, available from the BHS Bookshop.

Lesson 1 – Unmounted

(a) Training and test costs established with candidates and parents.

(b) Nominal roll call, test dates and training discussed.

(c) Application forms filled in – minimum age twelve years.

(d) Discover any problems candidates/horses may have.

(e) Issue books: the current editions of this Manual and the Highway Code.

(f) Correct dress for test, including checking hats.

(g) Show a road safety video or slides.

(h) Question and answer period, or papers taken home.

Lesson 2 – Unmounted. Off-road simulated road junction.

(a) Re-cap Lesson 1. Explain, demonstrate and practise (b)-(f).

(b) Observation and signals.

(c) Move-off from the side of the road.

(d) Correct positioning for left turns, major to minor, minor to major.

(e) Correct positioning for right turns, major to minor, minor to major.

(f) Dismount, lead and remount.

(g) Question paper.

Lesson 3 – Mounted. An assistant is useful. Parents attending.

(a) Check tack and hats.

(b) Re-cap previous lessons, practise mounted.

(c) Dismount, lead in-hand and remount.

(d) Traffic lights.

(e) Question paper.

Lesson 4 – Mounted. Off-road simulated road junctions.

(a) Check tack and hats.

(b) Re-cap previous lessons.

(c) Left and right turns, major to minor, minor to major.

(d) Traffic lights.

(e) Dismount, lead in-hand, remount.

(f) Link several manoeuvres.

(g) Question paper.

Lesson 5 – Mounted.

(a) Check tack and hats.

(b) Re-cap previous lessons.

(c) Traffic lights, left and right turns.

(d) Dismounting, leading and remounting.

(e) Staggered junctions.

(f) Zebra crossings.

(g) Related manoeuvres.

(h) Question papers.

Lesson 6 – Initially unmounted, horses present.

(a) Issue maps of routes.

(b) Walk the road route on foot.

(c) Mock test.

(d) Issue timetable to candidates (and parents if applicable) for the test day and brief candidates (and parents if applicable) on test-day procedure.

Sample theory questions

N.B. The traffic signs used on the following pages are © Crown copyright

1. What does a flashing amber light at a pelican crossing mean?

    a. You may proceed.

    b. You may proceed if there are no pedestrians on the crossing.

    c. You must stop.

2. When riding in snow, what would you do to improve your horse's footing?

    a. Dismount and lead your horse.

    b. Smear inside of hooves with grease.

    c. Ride in the middle of the road, putting grit down.

3. Which is the sign for one-way traffic?

    a. White arrow on a blue disc.

    b. White arrow on a blue rectangle.

    c. White and red arrows on a blue rectangle.

4. When you approach a zebra crossing, by law, when must you stop?

    a. At all times.

    b. When a pedestrian is approaching a crossing.

    c. When a pedestrian has at least one foot on the crossing.

5. If the road is narrow or has bends, how should a number of riders proceed?

    a. In pairs.

    b. No more than three abreast.

    c. In single file.

6. At traffic lights, which light or lights follow amber on its own?

    a. Green.

    b. Red.

    c. Red and amber.

7. You have to exercise your pony on the roads for an hour each day before 9 am. The rural rush hour is from 8 am to 9 am. Should you:

    a. Start your ride before 8 am?

    b. Ride between 8 am and 9 am?

    c. Ride between 7 am and 8 am when the light permits?

8. When negotiating roundabouts, what course would you take?

    a. The same route as a motor vehicle.

    b. Middle of the middle lane.

    c. To the left or near side.

9. Horse riders on the road:

a. Are a special case?

b. Unlike other traffic, are permitted to use bus lanes?

c. Have the same rights and responsibilities as other road users?

10. You should always wear a hard hat when riding, especially when on the road. Give the numbers and name the marks awarded to hats meeting the required BSI safety standard.

a. ....

b. ....

11. According to the Highway Code, are you allowed to ride or lead a horse or pony on a footpath or pavement?

a. Yes.

b. No.

c. Sometimes.

12. When approaching a frightening object at the side of the road, should the rider:

a. Use the left rein as the horse begins to shy?

b. Use the right rein before the horse begins to shy?

c. Use the right rein and right leg before the horse begins to shy?

13. At traffic lights, what does the colour amber on its own mean?

a. Get ready to stop.

b. Get ready to go.

c. Stop.

14. When riding in a party divided into groups, what distance should there be between them?

a. 30m (100ft).

b. 9m (30ft).

c. 15m (50ft).

15. Which is the road sign for STOP AND GIVE WAY?

16. If you are going to collect your horse from the paddock and ride him home on the road, would you:

a. Take a headcollar?

b. Take a saddle and bridle?

c. Take a bridle?

17. You are riding along a major road and wish to turn right into a minor road. A stream of traffic is approaching. Where would you stop and wait until the traffic had passed?

a. On the left of the major road, near the kerb or verge, opposite your new intended route.

b. Just left of the centre line on the major road, opposite your intended route on the minor road.

c. On the left of the major road, before the junction at the minor road.

18. If a car in front of you has one or more white lights shining to the rear, which way would you expect it to move?

a. Forwards.

b. Backwards.

c. Turning.

19. A rider should always wear a well-fitting hard hat when riding. Should it:

a. Have a BSI kite mark?

b. Have a slot for a picture of your horse?

c. Have a mackintosh cover?

20. According to the Highway Code, if you must ride at night or in murky weather, what kind of clothing is safest?

a. White.

b. Fluorescent.

c. Reflective.

21. Place the following in order of importance for a rider wishing to carry out an overtaking manoeuvre:

a. Signal.

b. Observe.

c. Manoeuvre.

 a. **b.** **c.**

22. At traffic lights, what colour, or combination of colours, follows green?

a. Amber.

b. Red and amber.

c. Green and amber.

23. When riding in a group on the road, what is the ideal distance that should be kept between horses?

a. Half a horse's length.

b. A horse's length.

c. Two horses' lengths.

24. Describe the road sign for ROAD WORKS:

a. Rectangular, white background, red border, black silhouette of man shovelling grit.

b. Triangular, white background, red border, black silhouette of man shovelling grit.

c. Triangular, red background, white border, black silhouette of man shovelling grit.

25. Are you permitted to ride on ornamental grass verges or central reservations?

a. Yes.

b. No.

c. Sometimes.

26. What is a rider required to do at a road junction where there is a continuous thick white line across the carriageway?

a. Stop at the STOP AND GIVE WAY sign.

b. Give way to traffic on the major road.

c. Stop and give way at the white line.

27. Where should novice riders/horses be positioned in a group of riders?

a. On the outside to give experience of traffic.

b. On the inside, middle of the group.

c. On the inside, at the front of the group.

28. What is the minimum form of insurance that every rider should have?

a. Fire and theft.

b. Personal accident.

c. Personal liability.

29. What is the first movement you should make before overtaking a parked vehicle or other obstruction?

a. Signal.

b. Look all around.

c. Change the whip to the inside hand.

30. What is the sequence of traffic lights, starting from red?

a. Red.

b. Green.

c. Red.

d. Red and amber.

e. Amber.

31. According to the Highway Code, where must you never ride or lead a horse?

a. Footpath or pavement.

b. Common land.

c. In a one-way street.

32. A rider must always wear a hard hat, approved to the BSI Standard. How should it be secured?

a. With a scarf.

b. With a two-point harness.

c. With a three-point harness.

33. What is the usual shape of road signs giving orders?

a. Circular.

b. Triangular.

c. Rectangular.

34. How should a horse and rider negotiate a roundabout?

a. Choose the proper lane for the exit.

b. Keep to the left.

c. Horses and riders should never use roundabouts.

35. If you are leading a horse either mounted or dismounted, where should you be positioned on the road?

a. On the left of the road, between the led horse and the traffic.

b. Facing oncoming traffic with you or the ridden horse nearest the verge.

c. On the left with the led horse between you and the traffic.

36. What is the procedure for crossing a main road when riding alone?

a. Look left, right, left again and cross quickly.

b. Wait for a break in the traffic, then cross quickly.

c. Look right, left, right again, behind and cross when the road is clear.

37. A riding hat should fit snugly on the head. If fitted, should the drawstring be:

a. Undone?

b. As tight as can be?

c. Adjusted to ensure a cushion of air between the top of your head and the hat?

38. What is a rider required to do at a road junction where there is a double row of broken white lines across the carriageway?

a. Stop at the STOP AND GIVE WAY sign.

b. Give way to traffic on the major road.

c. Continue, as road signs do not affect riders.

39. What shape is a road sign giving information?

a. Circular.

b. Rectangular.

c. Triangular.

40. What does a green traffic light mean?

a. Go.

b. Get ready to go.

c. Go only if it is safe to do so.

41. If you can foresee a dangerous road hazard, what is the best action?

a. Ride on the pavement.

b. Make the horse face up to it.

c. Make a detour to avoid the hazard.

42. When riding your horse/pony on the roads, are you required to obey all traffic signs and police signals?

a. Only those which relate to horse riders.

b. All traffic signs and police signals must be obeyed.

c. No, they do not relate to horse riders.

43. If the road is icy, what precautions should a rider take?

a. Ride the horse with a tight rein.

b. Quit the stirrup irons.

c. Shorten the stirrup leathers.

44. There is one eight-sided road sign – what does it tell you?

a. One-way street ahead.

b. Roundabout ahead.

c. Stop and give way.

45. You are waiting to turn at a junction. A car on the major road is signalling to turn left into your road. Should you:

a. Carry on with you turn?

b. Wait until the road is clear?

c. Wave him on?

46. What road marking would you expect to find when you have to give way to traffic when joining a major road?

a. Single broken white line across the carriageway.

b. Single continuous white line across the carriageway.

c. Double broken white lines across the carriageway.

47. Triangular signs with white background, and red borders:

a. Give orders?

b. Give information?

c. Give warnings?

48. What does the Highway Code direct that you must be able to do before riding your horse on the road?

a. Be used to riding in traffic.

b. The horse is used to traffic.

c. You can control your horse.

49. According to the Highway Code, if you are riding a horse on the public highway after dark, what should you wear?

a. A flashing amber light.

b. A reflector on the back of your hard hat.

c. A light showing white to the front, red to the rear.

50. At traffic lights, what colour follows amber on its own?

a. Green.

b. Red.

c. Red and amber.

51. A policeman or traffic warden on duty puts his hand up with the palm towards you, what must you do?

a. Wave back.

b. Dismount.

c. Stop.

52. When riding past a hazard on the side of the road, which is safest?

a. Bend the horse's head towards the hazard.

b. Bend the horse's head away from the hazard.

c. Keep his head straight.

53. What should a rider always carry in his pocket?

a. A penknife.

b. String.

c. A folding hoof-pick.

d. All of the above.

54. What is the principal reason why you, as a rider, should avoid trotting round corners/bends in the road?

a. To avoid tiring the horse.

b. The road surface may be very slippery.

c. To avoid stressing the horse's legs.

55. How is a party of riders advised to cross a main road?

a. Each rider to cross individually, each making his own judgment.

b. Cross in pairs, leading rider to make the decision when to cross.

c. Wait until all riders can cross the road together without leaving anyone behind.

56. If on a bridlepath you meet pedestrians coming towards you, would you:

a. Walk past slowly?

b. Dismount and lead your horse past?

c. Ignore them?

57. Place the following advice in order of importance:

a. Ride in company.

b. Try to avoid main roads.

c. Tell a responsible person your proposed route.

58. As a member of the BHS or the Pony Club, are you automatically covered at all times for third party legal liability insurance when riding?

a. Yes.

b. No.

c. Under certain circumstances.

59. What position on the road would you adopt if you were taking the third exit at a roundabout?

a. Cut across the central island.

b. On the right of the road.

c. On the left of the road.

60. A friend has fallen from her horse, which you have to lead home from your horse. The led horse wears a running martingale. How would you prepare him to be led?

61. What is the most important item to check on the horse before going out on the road?

a. His coat should gleam.

b. His shoes and hooves should be in good condition.

c. Hooves should be oiled.

62. Tick three items of importance that the rider should wear:

a. Riding hat to BSI standard.

b. Tie.

c. Jodhpurs.

d. Long-soled boots with a heel.

e. Hacking jacket.

f. Fluorescent/reflective tabard.

63. Tick three items of importance for the horse to wear before going out on the road:

a. Saddle.

b. Numnah.

c. Brushing boots.

d. Bridle.

e. Fluorescent/reflective leg bands.

f. Coloured browband.

64. When would a group of riders ride in single file?

a. On a major road.

b. Approaching a road junction.

c. On a narrow road.

65. Which three of the following items does the Highway Code stipulate when riding at night on the road?

a. Stirrup lamp.

b. Blinkers on the horse.

c. Torch.

d. Riding on verges.

e. Dismount and lead.

f. Reflective clothing.

g. Reflective leg bands.

66. If you are riding a horse and leading another, the led horse should be on your:

a. Left?

b. Right?

c. Behind you?

67. If your horse continually slips on an icy or slippery road, what action should you take?

a. Hope for the best.

b. Quit your irons and ride near to the verge/kerb.

c. Trot on to get clear of the problem as soon as possible.

68. A party of thirty-two riders wish to proceed on the public highway. What is the maximum number who should proceed as a group on the road?

a. The lot.

b. Groups of sixteen.

c. Groups of five.

d. Groups of eight.

69. Which sign means 'One-way traffic'?

a.   **b.**   **c.**

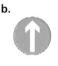

70. At a level crossing, the barriers come down, with the lights flashing and bells ringing. What should you do?

a. Cross as quickly as possible.

b. Stop in good time before the barrier.

c. Dismount.

71. Name three rules from the courtesy code.

72. You have a young/nervous horse, unused to traffic. Would you take him out alone?

a. Yes, he must learn to be bold.

b. No, go out in company to build his confidence.

c. No, never take him out of the box.

73. Where should a rider's hands be when overtaking an obstruction/hazard on the side of the road?

a. On the reins.

b. Signalling.

c. On the end of your arms.

74. If you keep your horse at grass a distance from home and you need a bucket of food with which to catch him, would you:

a. Take the bucket and feed with you from home and ride back with the bucket on your arm?

b. Leave the bucket in the field?

c. Take the feed down in your pocket to catch your horse?

75. What should you always do when a driver or other road user has been helpful and considerate to you as a rider?

a. Ride on.

b. Get out of his way.

c. Smile at him to acknowledge his courtesy.

76. A very noisy machine is in use at the side of the road. What should you do?

a. Keep going, urging your horse on.

b. Ask the operator to switch off the machine. Ride past thanking him.

c. Switch on your walkman.

77. Some train level crossings with no gates have amber lights followed by flashing red lights. When the amber lights are showing, should you:

a. Hurry across before the train comes?

b. Wait until all the lights go out, then cross?

c. Consult a railway timetable?

78. When riding behind a slow-moving car at the approach to a cross-roads, the driver makes an anti-clockwise circular movement with his right hand and arm. What is he signalling to other road users?

a. You are to overtake him.

b. He is turning right.

c. He is turning left.

79. On which one of the following can you ride or lead?

a. Motorway.

b. Footpath.

c. Bridleway.

80. At a pelican crossing does flashing amber mean?

a. Stop.

b. Move off.

c. Move off only if the crossing is clear of pedestrians.

81. Which footwear is ideal for riding?

a. Trainers.

b. Riding boots with through soles.

c. Wellingtons.

82. Which of the following describes the sign for NO ENTRY:

a. Horizontal red bar on a white disc?

b. Horizontal white bar on a red disc?

c. Horizontal white bar on a blue disc?

83. Which is the most important reason for walking your horse round a corner?

a. In case you meet something.

b. To give your horse a chance to see where he is going.

c. Because the road surface is often slippery.

84. Name the legislation under which young people are required to wear hard hats on the road.

85. Under legislation which has been in place since 1992, at what age are young people required to wear hard hats when riding on the road?

a. Up to ten years.

b. Up to fourteen years.

c. Up to eighteen years.

86. There is some headgear which is acceptable under the recent legislation concerning hard hats for young people when riding on the road but which is not acceptable to the British Horse Society. It is:

a. Polo helmets?

b. Pedal cycle helmets?

c. Jockey skull caps?

87. You are on your horse and waiting to turn right into a minor road from a major road. The headlights from an oncoming car flash twice. What does this mean according to the Highway Code?

a. It doesn't mean anything.

b. Get out of my way.

c. I am here.

d. You may turn across.

88. What is the meaning of this road sign?

a. Series of bends.

b. Double bend.

c. Slip road to motorway.

89. What is the meaning of this road sign?

a. Footpath only.

b. Pedestrian crossing.

c. Footpath end.

90. As a horse rider, how can you request a driver to stop?

   a. By calling out to him.

   b. By holding your hand up and out.

   c. By giving the slowing-down signal.

91. What does this road marking mean?

   a. Parking zone.

   b. Warning of 'Give Way' junction ahead.

   c. Traffic island.

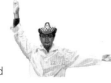

92. At a pelican crossing, what colour light do you see, as a road user, when the green man is flashing for pedestrians?

   a. Red.

   b. Flashing amber.

   c. Green.

93. What is the meaning of this road sign?

   a. Sharp deviation.

   b. Petrol station ahead.

   c. Count-down markers.

94. What does this signal, given by a police officer, mean?

   a. Stop, to traffic from the front.

   b. Stop, to traffic from behind.

   c. Stop, to traffic from the front and behind.

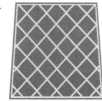

95. What is the meaning of this road marking?

   a. School, keep clear.

   b. Do not enter the marked area unless your exit is clear.

   c. Superstore car parking ahead.

96. When you are riding along the highway, in which hand should you carry your whip?

   a. It depends whether you're left-handed or right-handed.

   b. The left hand.

   c. The right hand.

97. As a horse rider, can you proceed past this road sign?

   a. On foot only.

   b. Yes.

   c. No.

98. What does this road sign mean?

   a. Accident ahead.

   b. Slippery road.

   c. Beware of drunken drivers.

99. Which of the following is not a current British Standard for protective headgear for horse riders?

   a. PAS 015.

   b. BS EN 1384.

   c. BS 6473.

100. What does this road marking mean?

   a. Give way to traffic on a major road.

   b. Give way to pedestrians.

   c. Stop until the green light shows.

101. What is the meaning of this road sign?

   a. Level crossing without a barrier.

   b. Cross roads ahead.

   c. No waiting.

102. What is the meaning of this road sign?

   a. T-junction.

   b. Dead end to the right.

   c. No heavy goods vehicles.

103. This road sign means that the national speed limit applies. What is the maximum national speed limit on a single carriageway road?

   a. 80mph.

   b. 70mph.

   c. 60mph.

104. When may equestrians ride on cycle paths?

a. During the rush-hour only.

b. At weekends only.

c. Never.

105. What is the meaning of this road sign?

a. Pony Club camp.

b. Parking place.

c. Press entrance.

106. What is the meaning of this road sign?

a. Gated level crossing.

b. Cattle market ahead.

c. School gates.

107. What does this road marking mean?

a. Centre line.

b. No overtaking or crossing at any time.

c. Hazard warning line.

108. What do the zig-zag lines on the approach to a zebra crossing mean?

a. Do not wait or park on the zig-zags.

b. Pedestrians may be crossing on the zig-zags.

c. Keep clear of lines when pedestrians are crossing.

109. What is the meaning of this road sign?

a. Slippery road.

b. Double bend.

c. Overhead electric cables.

110. Which of the following statements is the law's demand?

a. You must not ride a horse on the highway unless you have passed the Riding and Road Safety Test.

b. You must not wilfully ride a horse on the footpath.

c. You must not ride a horse under the age of four on public roads.

111. What is the meaning of this road sign?

a. Forestry Commission.

b. Christmas shoppers' parking.

c. Wild animals.

112. It is estimated that eight road accidents involving horses occur each day in the UK. In almost fifty per cent of these accidents, horses are struck from:

a. The rear?

b. The side?

c. The front?

113. Which of these road signs means T-junction?

a.   **b.**   **c.**

114. Which of these road signs warn of cattle?

a.   **b.**   **c.**

115. What does this road sign mean?

a. Concealed entrance to driveway.

b. Level crossing without barrier.

c. Cross-roads ahead.

116. What does this road marking mean?

a. One-way traffic only.

b. Mini roundabout.

c. Turning area.

117. What is the meaning of this road sign?

a. No horse riding.

b. Horse riders only.

c. Accompanied horses.

118. What wording is missing from this road sign? Is it:

a. NO ENTRY?

b. STOP?

c. ROUNDABOUT?

119. Which of the following white lines would you see across the roadway if there is a GIVE WAY sign before a major road?

a.

b.

c.

120. Approximately how many road accidents involving horses occur annually in the UK, according to BHS estimates?

a. 800.

b. 1280.

c. 3000.

121. What is the meaning of this road sign?

a. Gas leak.

b. Other danger.

c. Other hazard.

122. What is the meaning of this road sign?

a. T-junction.

b. No through road.

c. Traffic merges from the right.

123. What does this driver's arm signal mean to you as a horse rider?

a. You may overtake me.

b. I intend to move into the left or turn left.

c. I am going to slow down.

124. What is the meaning of this road sign?

a. Loose chippings.

b. Beware! Landslide.

c. Excessive spray.

125. The road you want to ride down has this road sign at its entrance. Would you:

a. Proceed, whilst watching out for buses approaching.

b. Find another route.

c. Proceed only if the light signal shows green.

126. What is the meaning of this road sign?

a. Pass either side.

b. Keep left unless turning right.

c. Centre lane closed.

Side-saddle candidates will receive additional sheets to include: positioning for maximum visibility on the road/at junctions/approaching hazards/dismount, leading and remount.

Answers to theory questions

1. b
2. b
3. b
4. c
5. c
6. b
7. c
8. c
9. c
10. BS EN 1384 (97), PAS 015 (94)
11. b
12. c
13. c
14. a
15. a
16. b
17. a
18. b
19. a
20. c
21. b, a, c
22. a
23. a
24. b
25. b
26. c
27. b
28. c
29. b
30. a, d, b, e, c
31. a
32. c
33. a
34. b
35. a
36. c
37. c
38. b
39. b
40. c
41. c
42. b
43. b
44. c

45. b
46. c
47. c
48. c
49. c
50. b
51. c
52. b
53. d
54. b
55. c
56. a
57. c, b, a
58. c
59. c
60. Tie martingale up, pass reins through bit to right side.
61. b
62. a, d, f
63. a, d, e
64. c
65. a, f, g
66. a
67. b
68. d
69. a
70. b
71. Consideration, good manners, acknowledgement.
72. b
73. a
74. b
75. c
76. b
77. b
78. c
79. c
80. c
81. b
82. b
83. c
84. Horses (Protective Head-gear for Young Riders) Regulations 1992.

85. b
86. b
87. c
88. b
89. b
90. b
91. b
92. b
93. a
94. c
95. b
96. c
97. b
98. b
99. c
100. a
101. a
102. a
103. c
104. c
105. b
106. a
107. c
108. a
109. c
110. b
111. c
112. a
113. a
114. b
115. c
116. b
117. c
118. b
119. b
120. c
121. b
122. c
123. b
124. a
125. b
126. a

INDEX

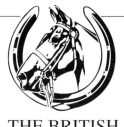

THE BRITISH
HORSE SOCIETY

Membership Application Form

Why not take advantage of British Horse Society Membership? The British Horse Society works for the well-being of all horses and ponies. If you would like to help us and yourself the best way is to join the Society. If you are already a member why not persuade a friend to join. Simply fill in the form below and return it with the first year's subscription.

Help us ensure that it is safe for you and your animals to be out and about by joining the B.H.S.

21 years of age and over
FULL ADULT MEMBERS   £33.50
*JOINING FEE
(also payable if
rejoining)   £5.00
     TOTAL   £38.50

Under 21 years of age
FULL JUNIOR
MEMBERSHIP   TOTAL   £25.00

ᴬThe joining fee is not applicable to Full Junior Members or applicants aged 60 or over providing the date of birth is included on the application form.

Cheques or Postal Orders should be made payable to:
The British Horse Society and sent with this application form.

Please use BLOCK CAPITALS

Name ....

Address ....

....

....

....

Post Code ....

Date of birth ....
(required if applying for Full Junior Membership or if applicants are aged 60 years or over.)

Signature ....

Tel No ....

Return your application form to Membership Department, British Horse Society, British Equestrian Centre, Kenilworth, Warwickshire CV8 2LR. Telephone Coventry (01203) 696697

Please help us enrol more members!

(Prices correct at time of publication)

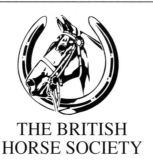

THE BRITISH
HORSE SOCIETY

BRITISH HORSE SOCIETY

RIDING AND ROAD SAFETY TEST

APPLICATION AND ENROLMENT FORM
(minimum age: 12 years)
(maximum age: 70 years)
(return to the BHS Regional/County Road Safety Representative as applicable)

Name ....

Address ....

....

Telephone no: .... Date of birth ....

Are you a member of the British Horse Society? ....

number ....

Are you a member of a Riding Club or the Pony Club? ....

If so, which Branch? ....

Address ....

Do you own a horse/pony? ....

If yes, where is the animal stabled or kept? ....

....

Do you attend a riding school? ....

If yes, where? ....

PARENT'S CONSENT FORM (for candidates under 16 years)

I hereby give approval for ....
to undertake the British Horse Society Road Safety Course and Test and agree
that the British Horse Society and its officers and employers shall not be under
any liability for any injury, damage or loss whatsoever and however caused.

I agree to pay .... per training session and *£10.00/£15.00 for the test to
cover all test costs.

*please delete as applicable (prices correct at time of publishing)

Date .... Parent's signature ....

Confidential
Form RS03

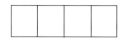

THE BRITISH HORSE SOCIETY
ACCIDENT REPORT

By completing this form you will help in putting together much needed statistics on horse-related traffic accidents, of which there are at least eight each day. The figure may be greater than this. This is necessary as the police accident form makes no provision for accurate recording of horse-related traffic accidents. Your contribution to our statistics will help to improve on that situation.

If more than one horse or rider involved please complete a separate form for each and staple them together

Date of accident:　　day of week ☐ 1　　date ☐☐　month ☐☐ 2　year ☐☐ 3

Time to the nearest hour:　　☐ a.m. 4　or　☐ p.m.

Town/Village/District: _____ **County:** _____ 5

ENTER NUMBERS OF EACH TYPE OF ROAD USER INVOLVED IN APPROPRIATE BOXES:

6.　Those involved:

horse	rider	pedestrian	pedal cycle	motor cycle	car/van	farm machinery
☐ 1	☐ 2	☐ 3	☐ 4	☐ 5	☐ 6	☐ 7

lorry	bus/coach	not known	other			
☐ 8	☐ 9	☐	☐ 10　specify _____			

TICK ONLY ONE MOST APPROPRIATE BOX FOR EACH OF THE FOLLOWING QUESTIONS:

7.　Was the horse:

ridden	led by walker	led by rider	loose	in harness	not known
☐ 1	☐ 2	☐ 3	☐ 4	☐ 5	☐

other ☐ 6　specify _____

8.　Was the rider:

alone	with one other horse	wih a group of horses (more than 2)	not known	no rider involved
☐ 1	☐ 2	☐ 3	☐	☐ 4 *(if no rider involved go to question 16)*

9.　Was rider wearing a hard hat:

no	yes	not known	
☐ 1	☐ 2	☐	*(if rider was not wearing a hard hat go to question 13)*

10.　Was hat displaced during the accident:

no	yes	not known
☐ 1	☐ 2	☐

11.　Was the hat:

BSI 3686	BSI 4472	BSI 6473	not known	other
☐ 1	☐ 2	☐ 3	☐	☐ 5　specify _____

12. How was the hat secured:

no strap/harness	elastic strap	simple chinstrap	harness	harness & chinstrap	not known
☐ 1	☐ 2	☐ 3	☐ 4	☐ 5	☐

☐ 7 other   specify _____

13. Did rider or horse fall:

neither fell	rider fell	horse fell	both fell	not known
☐ 1	☐ 2	☐ 3	☐ 4	☐

14. Was the rider:

not injured	injured	killed	not known
☐ 1	☐ 2	☐ 3	☐

15. Did the rider consult a:

GP/Doctor	hospital	none	not known
☐ 1	☐ 2	☐ 3	☐

16. Was/were other road user(s):

not injured	injured	killed	not known
☐ 1	☐ 2	☐ 3	☐

no other road users involved

☐ 4   *(if no other road users involved answer question 18 go to question 21*

17. Did the other road user(s) consult a:

GP/Doctor	hospital	none	not known
☐ 1	☐ 2	☐ 3	☐

18. Was the horse:

not injured	injured	killed	not known
☐ 1	☐ 2	☐ 3	☐

19. Which part of horse did vehicle hit:

front	side	behind	not known	no collision
☐ 1	☐ 2	☐ 3	☐	☐ 4

☐ 5 other   specify _____

20. Was the vehicle damaged:

no	not serious	serious	not known
☐ 1	☐ 2	☐ 3	☐

21. Age of rider:

under 12	12–16	19–30	31–64	65+	not known	no rider involved
☐ 1	☐ 2	☐ 3	☐ 4	☐ 5	☐	☐ 6

22. Sex of rider:

male	female	not known	no rider involved
☐ 1	☐ 2	☐	☐ 3

23. Type of area:

city	town	suburb	village	countryside	not known
☐ 1	☐ 2	☐ 3	☐ 4	☐ 5	☐

24. Type of road:

dual carriageway	main	minor	not known	not on road
☐ 1	☐ 2	☐ 3	☐	☐ 4

25. Which of the following statements best describes the accident:

Horse shied from shadow, bird etc and was hit by vehicle(s).. ☐ 1
Horse frightened by one vehicle and hit by other(s)... ☐ 2
Horse frightened and hit by same vehicle(s) .... ☐ 3
Horse frightened by vehicle(s) but not hit... ☐ 4
Horse shied from shadow, bird etc and not hit by vehicle(s).................................. ☐ 5
No vehicle involved.. ☐ 6
Details not known .... ☐
Horse escaped into traffic and hit by vehicle(s)... ☐ 8
Other (please specify) .... ☐ 7

Give brief details of accident:

_____

_____

_____

_____

26. In what capacity are you filling in this form:

rider	motorist	witness	friend	police	relative
☐ 1	☐ 2	☐ 3	☐ 4	☐ 5	☐ 6

other

☐ 7   specify _____

A representative of the British Horse Society may wish to obtain more details about this accident:

Your name: _____

Your address:
PLEASE PRINT _____

_____

_____

Telephone No: daytime _____ evening _____

Please complete and send to:

BRITISH HORSE SOCIETY
ROAD SAFETY DEPT
BRITISH EQUESTRIAN CENTRE
STONELEIGH PARK, KENILWORTH
WARWICKSHIRE CV8 2LR

YOUR NAME AND ADDRESS WILL NOT BE ENTERED INTO THE COMPUTER

Thank you for completing this form.